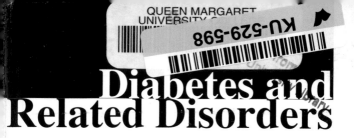

Diabetes and Related Disorders

Stuart Ross MB ChB, FRACP, FRCP(C)
Endocrinologist and Clinical Professor of Medicine
University of Calgary, Alberta, Canada

Roger Gadsby BSc, MB ChB, DCH, DRCOG, FRCGP
General Practitioner and Senior Lecturer in Primary Care
University of Warwick, Warwick, UK

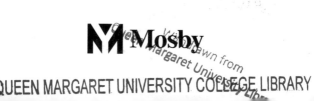

M Mosby

Acknowledgement

The authors wish to thank Ann Stringer for her help in the preparation of this book.

MOSBY
An imprint of Elsevier Limited.

© 2004 Elsevier Limited.

The Publisher's policy is to use paper manufactured from sustainable forests

M Mosby is a registered trademark of Elsevier Limited.

ISBN 0-7234-3317-8

Cataloguing in Publication Data
Catalogue records for this book are available from the US Library of Congress and the British Library.

Note
Medical knowledge is constantly changing. As new information becomes available, changes in treatment, procedures, equipment and the use of drugs become necessary. The authors and the publishers have taken care to ensure that the information given in this text is accurate and up to date. However, readers are strongly advised to confirm that the information, especially with regard to drug usage, complies with the latest legislation and standards of practice. Website addresses correct at time of going to press.

Printed in China.

Contents

Abbreviations

ACE	angiotensin converting enzyme
AIIRA	angiotensin II receptor antagonist
BMI	body mass index
CHD	coronary heart disease
DKA	diabetic ketoacidosis
ECG	electrocardiogram
GDM	gestational diabetes mellitus
HDL	high density lipoprotein
HHS	hyperosmolar, hyperglycaemic state
HONK	hyperosmolar, non-ketotic coma
IDDM	insulin dependent diabetes mellitus
IFG	impaired fasting glucose
IGT	impaired glucose tolerance
IRMA	intraretinal microvascular abnormalities
LDL	low density lipoprotein
NHS	National Health Service (UK)
NIDDM	non-insulin dependent diabetes mellitus
OGTT	oral glucose tolerance test
PAI-1	plasminogen activator inhibitor type 1
RCT	randomized controlled trial
TSH	thyroid stimulating hormone
TZDs	thiazolidinediones
WHO	World Health Organization

Introduction

Diabetes is a huge public health time-bomb that is exploding across the world. The number of people in the world with diabetes is expected to double in the 13-year period 1997 – 2010, leading to a predicted 221 million people with diabetes in the world by 2010.

Prevalence rates in Asian countries are expected to rise by over 100%, in Africa by 82%, in Europe by 51% and in North America by 35%. In many countries diabetes is now the leading cause of blindness in people of working age, and the leading cause of renal failure. Life expectancy is reduced by over 10 years in Type 2 diabetes, and over 75% of people with the condition will die of cardiovascular disease.

Diabetes complications are preventable. There is powerful evidence from long-term studies that good quality diabetes care can reduce the burden of the condition and its complications. Effective diabetes care can best be achieved by multidisciplinary teams of healthcare professionals offering straightforward interventions to everyone with diabetes and encouraging people living with diabetes to be empowered to control their condition themselves.

Management of diabetes also requires aggressive management of associated cardiovascular risk factors, such as hypertension and dyslipidaemia, that are frequently present in the patient with Type 2 diabetes.

This pocket textbook is designed to give readers the evidence and information to improve diabetes care. It is evidence based and fully referenced to enable readers to look up the primary sources. It is jointly written by a Canadian endocrinologist working in secondary care and a British general practitioner with a special interest in diabetes. It therefore gives insights into the condition from several different perspectives.

There are differences in emphasis in diabetes care in different countries of the world, with slightly differing targets and different terminologies. This book aims to be as inclusive as possible and to promote the concept that individualized treatment of the diabetic patient will provide an opportunity to improve the health and quality of life of the patient with diabetes.

We trust that this pocket textbook will be widely used to inform, assist and guide doctors and healthcare professionals around the world in their care of people with diabetes.

In the interests of consistency UK generic names have been used throughout this book. However, some alternative names used in other countries are listed below.

UK generic name	Alternative generic name
Soluble insulin	Human regular insulin
Isophane insulin	NPH insulin
Insulin zinc suspension	Insulin lente
Glibenclamide	Glyburide

Definition, classification and diagnosis

Definition

The term diabetes mellitus describes a metabolic disorder of multiple aetiology characterized by chronic hyperglycaemia with disturbances of carbohydrate, fat and protein metabolism resulting from defects in insulin secretion, insulin action or both.[1]

Several pathogenic processes are involved in the development of diabetes. These include processes that destroy the beta-cells of the pancreas with consequent insulin deficiency, and others that result in resistance to insulin action. The abnormalities of carbohydrate, fat and protein metabolism are due to deficient action of insulin on target tissues resulting from either insensitivity to, or lack of, insulin.

The long-term effects of diabetes include the progressive development of the specific microvascular complications of retinopathy (which can lead to blindness), nephropathy (which can develop to end-stage renal failure), and neuropathy (which can result in foot ulceration and amputation, erectile dysfunction and autonomic neuropathy). People with diabetes are also at an increased risk of cardiovascular, peripheral vascular and cerebrovascular disease. These macrovascular risks are so significant that Type 2 diabetes has been defined as "a condition of increased vascular risk associated with hyperglycaemia".

Classification

The recent WHO consultation[1] has recommended classifying diabetes into four groups: Type 1, Type 2, Other Specific Types (less common causes of diabetes where the underlying defect or disease process can be identified) and Gestational Diabetes (Table 1).

Diagnosing diabetes

New WHO criteria for diagnosing diabetes were adopted in 2000. Diabetes is now diagnosed as a fasting plasma glucose of 7 mmol/l and above (it was 7.8 mmol/l under the previous

Table 1. Aetiological classification of diabetes[1]

Type 1 (beta-cell destruction, usually leading to absolute insulin deficiency)
- autoimmune
- idiopathic

Type 2 (may range from predominantly insulin resistance with relative insulin deficiency to a predominantly secretory defect with or without insulin resistance)

Other specific types
- genetic defects of beta-cell function, e.g. maturity onset diabetes of young (MODY 1, 2 , 3 and 4)
- genetic defects of insulin action, e.g. Leprechaunism
- diseases of the exocrine pancreas, e.g. cystic fibrosis or haemachromatosis
- endocrinopathies, e.g. Cushings
- drug or chemical induced, e.g. steroids
- infections
- uncommon forms of immune-mediated diabetes
- other genetic syndromes sometimes associated with diabetes

Gestational diabetes

WHO diagnostic criteria). The blood glucose level for diagnosing diabetes with a random plasma glucose or a post 75 g glucose challenge of 11.1 mmol/l or above is unchanged from the previous diagnostic criteria.

Under these new criteria, those with fasting glucose levels below 6 mmol/l are classified as normal and those with levels between 6 and 7 mmol/l are classified as having impaired fasting glucose (IFG).

If IFG is diagnosed, it is recommended that an oral glucose tolerance test is performed.[2] If the 2 hour glucose level is 11.1 mmol/l or above diabetes is diagnosed. If the 2 hour level is below 7.8 mmol/l it is classified as normal, if it is between 7.8 and 11.1 mmol/l a diagnosis of impaired glucose tolerance (IGT) is made (Figures 1 and 2).

IGT and IFG are together now being called pre-diabetes.[3]

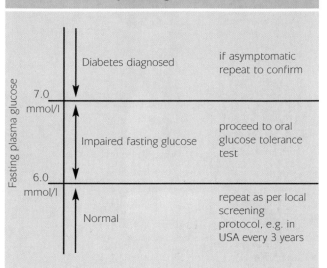

Figure 1. Diagnosis of diabetes using fasting plasma glucose

Fasting plasma glucose

Diabetes diagnosed — if asymptomatic repeat to confirm

7.0 mmol/l

Impaired fasting glucose — proceed to oral glucose tolerance test

6.0 mmol/l

Normal — repeat as per local screening protocol, e.g. in USA every 3 years

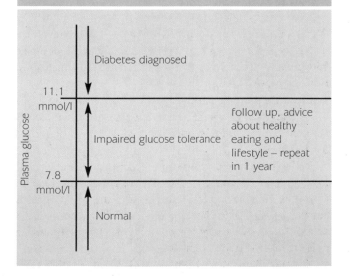

Figure 2. Diagnosis of diabetes using OGTT – plasma glucose 2 hours after a 75 g glucose load

Plasma glucose

Diabetes diagnosed

11.1 mmol/l

Impaired glucose tolerance — follow up, advice about healthy eating and lifestyle – repeat in 1 year

7.8 mmol/l

Normal

Pre-diabetes and evidence-based prevention of Type 2 diabetes

People who have IFG and/or IGT are at an intermediate stage of disordered carbohydrate metabolism. They have an increased risk of progressing to diabetes and macrovascular disease. People with IGT have a 50% 10-year risk of developing diabetes.[4] It is clear from several studies that lifestyle interventions with weight reduction and increased physical activity can prevent the development of diabetes in people at risk of developing the condition.

In a study from Finland, researchers took 522 middle-aged people known to have IGT, and divided them into a control and intervention group. The intervention group received individualized counselling for dietary change, weight loss and increased physical activity. The mean weight loss in the intervention group was 4.2 kg in the first year and 0.8 kg in the control group. The intervention group also increased their level of physical activity.

The cumulative incidence of diabetes after 4 years was 11% in the intervention group and 23% in the control group, a risk reduction of 58%.[5]

In the USA Diabetes Prevention Study, 3243 people with IGT or IFG were assigned either to placebo, metformin 850 mg twice daily or a lifestyle modification programme with the goals of at least a 7% weight loss and at least 150 minutes of physical activity per week. The average follow up was 2.8 years. Lifestyle intervention reduced the incidence of diabetes by 58% and metformin by 31% as compared with placebo.

The lifestyle intervention was systematic and intensive, with study participants receiving detailed individualized counselling. Fifty% of the participants in the lifestyle group achieved the weight loss target and 58% achieved the activity goal. The study was not designed to test the relative contributions of diet, weight loss and increased activity, and the effect of each of the components separately remains to be determined.[6]

This reduction of 58% by lifestyle intervention was exactly the same as in the Finnish study, and is far greater than that obtained by metformin therapy. The USA study used individualized support, the Finnish one used group support.

The problem with translating these impressive results into everyday clinical practice is that the interventions were expensive in both time and human resources. Most countries do not have the resources to deliver them at present and it is questionable whether such prevention will ever become politically important enough to have sufficient money and human resource allocated to it.

In another study of 1429 people with IGT, called the Stop-NIDDM study, the drug acarbose, along with lifestyle and exercise advice, was compared with placebo and advice. This agent delays the absorption of glucose in the gut and has the side effects of flatulence, abdominal cramps and diarrhoea, which make it difficult to tolerate.

The results showed a 36% reduction in the development of diabetes, but 30% had to discontinue the study, nearly half of them in the first few months. The most common single cause of early discontinuation was gastrointestinal side effects.[7]

Another approach to reducing the incidence of diabetes, which has been tested in an RCT, is to use the drug orlistat, which acts locally in the gut to reduce absorption of ingested fat, in combination with lifestyle change. In this Xendos study 3304 obese individuals, 21% of whom had IGT, were given lifestyle advice and either placebo or orlistat 120 mg three times daily, and were followed for 4 years. Those receiving orlistat lost on average 6.9 kg in weight against 4.1 kg on placebo. The cumulative incidence of Type 2 diabetes was 9% in the lifestyle plus placebo group and 6.2% in the lifestyle plus orlistat group, a risk reduction of 37%. This study shows that in an obese population in which 21% had IGT, orlistat plus lifestyle change over 4 years resulted in a greater weight loss and a significantly reduced incidence of Type 2 diabetes compared with intensive lifestyle changes alone. Orlistat was well tolerated in the study.[8]

The evidence from these four important RCTs is that diabetes can be prevented in people at significant risk of developing the condition. Lifestyle and exercise modification programmes work in research trials where there is considerable input of money and human resources, but there are concerns as to whether such lifestyle change can be introduced and maintained in normal clinical practice situations.

Diabetes symptoms

The classical symptoms of hyperglycaemia are polyuria and polydipsia. They commonly occur in people newly presenting with Type 1 diabetes and may be associated with weight loss, nausea, vomiting and dehydration when ketosis is occurring.

In Type 2 diabetes, symptoms may be absent, or may be very non-specific such as tiredness and lethargy. People and healthcare professionals may think that such non-specific symptoms reflect the normal ageing process and so the diagnosis of Type 2 diabetes may be overlooked. Campaigns to alert members of the general public to the symptoms of diabetes have been instituted in the UK and other countries.[9]

Healthcare professionals need to "think diabetes" whenever someone presents with non-specific symptoms, and to arrange blood glucose testing as appropriate.

Two abnormal glucose measurements need to be obtained in an asymptomatic person before a diagnosis of diabetes is made.[2]

The diagnosis of diabetes has important medico-legal implications and so diagnostic blood glucose estimations must be from a laboratory with appropriate quality control rather than handheld glucose oxidase stick testing measurements.

Type 1 diabetes: epidemiology and prevention

Type 1 diabetes usually presents with a short history (from a few days to a few weeks) of polyuria, polydipsia, and weight loss often accompanied by nausea, vomiting, abdominal pain and dehydration. The most common cause (of over 90% of cases) is autoimmune destruction of pancreatic beta-cells. The exact aetiology is not fully understood, but it is probable that environmental factors trigger the onset of Type 1 diabetes in individuals who have a genetic predisposition. The environmental factors involved have not been proven, but candidates that have been postulated include viruses, foodstuffs, and cows' milk protein.

Although Type 1 diabetes can occur at any age, it occurs most often in children and teenagers. There is a marked regional variation in the incidence of Type 1 diabetes around the world. North European countries such as Sweden and Finland show high frequencies of 30–35 cases per year per 100,000 population, whereas in Japan and China the incidence is nearer two cases per year per 100,000 population.

A number of countries keep detailed registers of young people with Type 1 diabetes, and in these countries the incidence of Type 1 diabetes is rising. Recent information from the UK suggests that in the under 16 age group rates have risen from 16.5 to 19 per 100,000 per year from 1991 to 1998. This study predicts that rates will rise to 30 per 100,000 per year by 2010.[10]

In most countries people with Type 1 diabetes make up around 10% of the total diabetes population of that country.

Preventing Type 1 diabetes

The concept of using agents to prevent the development of Type 1 diabetes in people deemed to be at high risk (e.g. people with autoimmune markers who are relatives of people with established Type 1 diabetes) are being tested in RCTs.

In the Diabetes Prevention Trial of Type 1 diabetes (DPT-1)[11] insulin was given by annual intravenous infusion as well as twice daily low-dose subcutaneous insulin. The cumulative incidence of diabetes was the same in this group as in the observational control group.

In the European Nicotinamide Diabetes Intervention Trial (ENDIT)[12] nicotinamide treatment did not reduce the risk of developing diabetes against placebo.

Type 2 diabetes: epidemiology, screening and prevention

Type 2 diabetes is typically diagnosed in middle aged or older people when they present with vague symptoms of ill health such as tiredness and lethargy. Many people with Type 2 diabetes are asymptomatic and the diagnosis is only made when they present for a routine medical examination or when they are admitted to hospital for an unrelated condition.

The recently published *Diabetes Atlas 2000*[13] estimates that there are currently around 151 million people in the age group 20–79 with diabetes in the world, a global prevalence of 4.6%. Worldwide the number of people with diabetes is expected to double over the 13-year period 1997 – 2010 to a total of 221 million. Prevalence rates are expected to rise by 111% in Asia, 93% in Africa, 51% in Europe and 35% in North America.[13]

In many developed countries over the past 100 years improved nutrition, better hygiene and the control of infectious disease has resulted in improved longevity. This has unmasked many age-related non-communicable diseases such as Type 2 diabetes. The term epidemiological transition has been used to describe this shift in disease patterns, which is now beginning to affect the developing countries.[14] It has catapulted Type 2 diabetes from a rare condition 100 years ago to its current position as a major global contributor to disability and death.

The major factors leading to this massive explosion in the numbers of people developing Type 2 diabetes are obesity and the increasingly sedentary lifestyle of many in the world. Type 2 diabetes is now being diagnosed in teenagers, most of whom are significantly obese. They are likely to manifest the serious complications of diabetes when they are in the 30 to 40 year old age range.[15]

Preventing Type 2 diabetes

There is clear evidence that individuals with impaired glucose tolerance can reduce their risk of developing Type 2 diabetes if they are helped to eat a balanced diet, lose weight and increase their levels of physical activity.[5,6]

Clearly levels of obesity and lack of physical activity are major public health issues in many developed and developing countries. They need to be tackled politically at population levels. However, healthcare workers also need to support individuals in weight reduction and increasing physical activity.

Screening for Type 2 diabetes

The value of population screening for Type 2 diabetes is an issue of debate, and policies vary between countries. For example, the American Diabetes Association recommends three yearly screening for all people in the USA over the age of 45. However, when this strategy was tested in a low diabetes risk Caucasian population in England, it was concluded that screening based on age alone was not cost-effective, but that screening of high-risk populations based on a combination of age, obesity, a positive family history, and hypertension was cost-effective.[16] Therefore, population-based screening for asymptomatic individuals is not currently recommended in England. A large epidemiology screening study in Canada, did, however, demonstrate benefit in screening patients above the age of 40 when both previously undetected diabetes and glucose intolerance were identified in 5.7% of the population.[17] A national screening programme targeting high-risk groups, for diabetes and cardiovascular disease, may be the way forward in developed countries.

Type 2 diabetes, the metabolic syndrome and insulin resistance

Insulin resistance, an insulin signalling defect is found in up to 25% of the general, apparently healthy population.[18] In 1988, Reaven postulated that the co-existence of risk factors, including dyslipidaemia, hypertension, obesity and Type 2 diabetes mellitus was due to the primary underlying pathology of insulin resistance.[18] He suggested that many individuals with insulin resistance remain non-diabetic because they are able to compensate for their insulin resistance by secreting more insulin (hyperinsulinaemia). In people liable to Type 2 diabetes, Reaven suggested that the beta-cell of the pancreas would eventually be unable to compensate, with the initial development of IGT followed by Type 2 diabetes. Thus both beta-cell dysfunction and insulin resistance are normally required for the development of Type 2 diabetes.

Other components have been added subsequently to the syndrome including hyperuricaemia, abnormalities of clotting factors and proteinuria/microalbuminuria.

Impact and cost of diabetes

Life expectancy is reduced, on average, by more than 20 years in people with Type 1 diabetes, and by up to 10 years in people with Type 2 diabetes.[19]

Mortality rates from cardiovascular disease are two to five times higher in patients with diabetes compared with non-diabetics. Around 80% of people with Type 2 diabetes will die of cardiovascular disease, many prematurely.[20]

In the UK, diabetes is the leading cause of renal failure, the second most common cause of lower limb amputation and the leading cause of blindness in people of working age.[19]

People with diabetes are twice as likely to be admitted to hospital as the general population and, once admitted, are likely to have a length of stay that is up to twice the average.[19]

In the UK, around 5% of total NHS financial resources and up to 10% of hospital inpatient resources are used for the care of people with diabetes.[14] The most recent cost data from the UK have increased these figures to 8% of total NHS spend, and this now mirrors that from the USA and Canada.[20,21]

Delivering diabetes care

Good diabetes care is not "rocket science". It involves doing simple things regularly and systematically, and recording the information. No single healthcare professional can do all the simple things required. Multidisciplinary teams of healthcare professionals working together and sharing information are required to deliver good diabetes care.

Evidence for models of care delivery

Reviews of the evidence for interventions to improve the management of diabetes in primary care, outpatient and community settings[22] and a meta-analysis of randomized controlled trials of general practice diabetes care[23] have been published. Although various methodological limitations were observed in the studies outlined in these reviews, important conclusions can be drawn.[24]

1. Complex professional interventions often improve the process of care, although most studies did not assess the effect on health-related outcomes.
2. Process improvements were seen in studies that included structured and regular review. A small beneficial effect in glycaemic control was seen in studies in which a nurse[25] or pharmacist[26] assumed part of the physician's role.
3. Features, which were associated with improvement in process measures, included computer-assisted recall and reminder systems, in combination with professional interventions.[27]
4. The involvement of nurses and the inclusion of patient education were associated with positive effects on patient outcomes.[28]

Conclusion

Combinations of professional interventions, organisational interventions, nurse involvement and patient education often do make a positive difference in the process of care and can make a positive difference to the outcome of care.[24] There is

Table 2. Protocol for annual review

Discussion

General health and well being, including life with diabetes, e.g. driving, etc

Glycaemic control including self-monitoring information and symptoms of hypo- or hyperglycaemia

Diabetes knowledge and self-management skills, including the importance of good metabolic control and healthy lifestyle

Specific enquiry about smoking and alcohol consumption, and level of physical activity

Specific enquiry about vision problems, chest pain, dyspnoea, intermittent claudication, neuropathy and erectile dysfunction

Examination

Weight, waist circumference and calculated body mass index

Blood pressure

Foot examination to include: footwear, condition of skin and nails, deformity and ulceration, foot pulses, sensitivity to 10g nylon monofilament

Insulin injection site inspection (if appropriate)

Investigations

Urinalysis for proteinuria by dipstick test – if negative send urine for microalbumunuria screening

Review of blood test results taken 1 or 2 weeks before to include: HbA_{1c}, creatinine, full lipid profile

Results from local diabetes retinopathy screening programme

Management

Optimize glycaemic therapy

Optimize blood pressure

Referral for further diet or exercise advice as necessary

Calculation of, and management of, CHD risk

Management of any long-term complications and referral to others as needed

Target setting with the patient for the next 12 months, agree review date

Recording

Ensure all results and findings are recorded on appropriate clinical record system and patient-held records thus an emerging evidence base for multidisciplinary diabetes care.

Monitoring for complications and multidisciplinary care

Every person with diabetes needs a comprehensive annual review to monitor control and check for complications. When control is suboptimal or where changes in therapy are being instigated and their effects monitored people may need to be seen much more frequently, perhaps every 3 months.

A suggested protocol for annual review is given in Table 2 and recommended outcome goals are given in Table 3.

Supporting self-management

Diabetes is a chronic life-long condition that impacts upon almost every aspect of life. Living with diabetes is not easy. Medication is usually self-administered, while lifestyle changes involving diet and physical exercise require commitment and active involvement. Those with Type 1 diabetes have to balance the risks of hypoglycaemia against the long-term danger of hyperglycaemia on a daily basis. Those with Type 2 diabetes usually need to change their lifestyle, which is difficult if the individual does not feel ill.

A diagnosis of diabetes can lead to poor psychological adjustment, including self-blame and denial, which can create barriers to effective self-management. The diagnosis can also create or reinforce a sense of low self-esteem and induce depression.

The provision of information, education and psychological support that facilitates self-management is therefore the cornerstone of diabetes care. People with diabetes need the knowledge, skills and motivation to assess their risks, to understand what they will gain from changing their behaviour or lifestyle and to act on that understanding by engaging in appropriate behaviours.[19]

Initial education at diagnosis, and continuing education is therefore vital. In many countries most people who are newly

Table 3. Goals for annual review

Glycaemic control
- Goal is HbA$_{1c}$ of 7% or below
- If person has established CHD a goal of 6.5% or below may be helpful
- If these goals are not desirable or practical because of other co-morbidities or other reasons, ANY reduction in HbA$_{1c}$ has clinical benefit in reducing adverse outcomes, so for example reducing HbA$_{1c}$ from 10.5% to 9.5% is worthwhile

Blood pressure
- Goal is 140/80 mmHg or below
- If person has any signs of nephropathy a target of 130/75 mmHg or below may be helpful
- If these goals are not desirable or practical because of other co-morbidities or other reasons, ANY reduction in blood pressure has benefit in reducing adverse outcomes, so for example reduction from 170/100 to 160/90 mmHg is worthwhile

Eyes
- Goal is to ensure that person has a yearly review by an approved diabetes retinopathy screening programme
- Referral for urgent laser treatment is needed if sight-threatening retinopathy is detected

Feet
- Goal is an annual foot examination to determine "at risk" status
- People with any signs of "at risk" feet need to be seen in a foot protection programme for further assessment and further preventive foot education
- Anyone presenting with newly developed ulceration and/or cellulites needs to be referred urgently to a multidisciplinary footcare team

CHD risk
- Goal is annual assessment and treatment with statin and low-dose aspirin where indicated

diagnosed with Type 1 diabetes will receive this initial education in the secondary care setting either in hospital or in a Diabetes Centre while most people with newly diagnosed Type 2 diabetes will receive initial education and care in the primary care setting.

The content of diabetes education

The International Diabetes Federation (IDF) has published International Consensus Standards of Practice for Diabetes Education[29] that outline the key elements and frameworks by which the structure, process and outcome of diabetes education can be assessed. The suggested content of diabetes self-management education from the Education Study Group of the European Association for the Study of Diabetes (EASD)[30] are outlined in Table 4.

Table 4. Self-management diabetes education programme content

A. Diabetes overview

B. Stress and psychological adjustment

C. Family involvement and social support

D. Nutrition

E. Exercise and activity

F. Medications

G. Monitoring and use of results

H. Relationship between nutrition, exercise, medication and blood glucose levels

J. Prevention, detection and treatment of chronic complications

K. Foot, skin and dental care

L. Behaviour change strategies, goal setting, risk factor reduction and problem solving

M. Benefits, risks and management options for improving glucose control

N. Preconception care, pregnancy and gestational diabetes

O. Use of healthcare systems and community resources

Method of diabetes education

The level and pace of learning varies between individuals, supplying too little information or inundating the person with too much information are equally disastrous. It helps to begin by asking about previous knowledge and experience of diabetes. Then any misconceptions about diabetes can be dealt with and a clear understanding of the basics of diabetes can be given.

Educating people newly diagnosed with Type 2 diabetes in small groups where peer support can be provided is becoming a popular method in some countries.

Using written materials and computer-based programmes

Education is enhanced if verbal education is backed up by written information. Many national diabetes organisations provide very helpful literature that can be used. Computer-assisted programmes that provide education and trigger self-management have also been shown to provide benefit in terms of both metabolic and psychosocial outcomes.[31]

Self-management: nutrition

The modern emphasis is away from the concept of the diabetic diet towards the concept of healthy eating. This concept of healthy eating is important for all the population and its adoption by all members of the family of the person newly diagnosed with Type 2 diabetes will be a great help in self-management.

A simple written guide as outlined in Table 5 can reinforce healthy eating messages until full assessment and more detailed education can be given by a trained dietician.

Self-management: physical activity and exercise

Encouraging physical activity and exercise in people with diabetes is an important part of self-management. It has been shown to help prevent the onset of Type 2 diabetes in people with IGT. It is important that advice should be realistic, simple, individualized and enjoyable. Walking for 20 to 30 minutes a day is a realistic goal for many people with diabetes.[32]

Table 5. A simple introduction to nutrition and diabetes

1. Eat regularly

- do not miss meals, aim to have three meals a day
- eat five portions of fruit and vegetables per day

2. Avoid added sugar and sugary foods

- do not add sugar to any food or drink, use artificial sweeteners instead
- avoid drinks sweetened with sugar, instead use low calorie and sugar-free drinks (often labelled as diet drinks)
- avoid sugary biscuits, cakes, sugary puddings or desserts, sweets and chocolates
- instead have fresh fruit for dessert

3. Eat plenty of fibre

- good sources are: fibre-rich breakfast cereals, whole-grain bread, oats, beans, lentils, fruit, vegetables, potatoes, brown rice, wholemeal pasta

4. Eat less fat

- use skimmed or semi-skimmed milk
- cut down on butter, margarine, oil, lard and cheese
- eat lean meat and remove visible fat
- grill food rather than frying it

5. Avoid special "diabetic" products

- they are often expensive

6. Try to be the right weight for your height

Self-management: coping with illness

Understanding and applying the "illness rules" are important in the self-management of minor illnesses in people with diabetes.[33] They are outlined in Table 6.

Supporting self-management in Type 1 diabetes

Historically many people newly diagnosed with Type 1 diabetes were admitted to hospital for education, and insulin initiation. The trend in most countries is now to educate and initiate insulin treatment on an outpatient basis whenever possible.

Table 6. Illness rules

- minor illness, e.g. colds and flu, may cause blood glucose levels to rise temporarily – it is important to monitor more frequently during illness
- continue to take diabetes medications (tablets and/or insulin)
- vomiting and diarrhoea may result in the loss of a lot of fluid – try to drink extra fluids, sipping small quantities at a time
- if you are not hungry, substitute solid meals with liquids or light diet, e.g. soups, milk, ice cream, etc
- it is safe to take paracetamol (acetaminophen) or other treatments to reduce high temperatures, and for headache and sore throat symptoms
- it is safe to take "sugar-free" cough remedies
- if vomiting or illness persist contact your doctor for further advice

In some parts of Germany people newly diagnosed with Type 1 diabetes receive initial education as inpatients as part of a structured programme. There is also evidence that such a 5 day programme can improve control in people with Type 1 diabetes who are poorly controlled.[34]

This work has formed the basis of the Dose Adjustment for Normal Eating (DAPHNE) programme in the UK. It is an outpatient education model that involves a structured training programme in intensive insulin therapy and self-management. People are taught to match their insulin dose to food intake on a meal-by-meal basis. The aim is to enable people to maintain healthy glycaemic control without an increased risk of severe hypoglycaemia and with minimal support from healthcare professionals.[35] The results show that the programme improves quality of life and glycaemic control without worsening severe hypoglycaemia or cardiovascular risk. The study authors conclude that the programme has the potential to enable more people to adopt intensive insulin treatment and is worthy of further investigation.

Monitoring diabetes control

Self-monitoring of capillary blood glucose by people with diabetes is possible using home monitoring devices. A small drop of blood is obtained by using a device for automatic finger pricking and is placed on a strip. The glucose in the sample can either cause a colour change in the strip, or may generate a current in the newer electrochemically based strips. The strip is then placed in a meter that gives a reading of the glucose concentration. Blood glucose monitoring technology is developing quickly and a number of new meters are being developed that require very small quantities of blood. This can enable blood samples to be taken from alternative sites such as the forearm, which are much less painful than the fingertip.

Some meters can now store the blood glucose results and export them to a home computer where the results can be shown graphically and be sent electronically to a healthcare professional for advice.

The literature on whether blood glucose monitoring improves control is difficult to assess. However, a comprehensive package of care that includes glucose self-monitoring is usually effective in improving glycaemic control in Type 1 diabetes.[31]

The place of blood glucose monitoring in people with Type 2 diabetes controlled on diet or oral therapy remains controversial. There is usually little scope for self-management therapy change in Type 2 diabetes and so the use of the much cheaper technology of monitoring urine glucose using strips is suggested by some healthcare professionals.

Monitoring glycaemic control using HbA_{1c} measurements

HbA_{1c} is a measure of the integrated blood glucose control over the preceding 2 to 3 months and is formed by the attachment of glucose to haemoglobin. It can be measured by several different laboratory methods, which may not give equivalent results. The two major glycaemic outcome studies in diabetes used the same measurement technique and so HbA_{1c}

measurements taken to assess glycaemic control need to be aligned to this DCCT/UKPDS assay.

Glycaemic targets in Type 1 diabetes

The Diabetes Control and Complications Trial (DCCT)[36] showed that an intensively controlled group of people with Type 1 diabetes with an average HbA_{1c} of 7%, had significantly reduced diabetes complications when compared with a normal treatment group whose HbA_{1c} averaged 9%. A level of HbA_{1c} of 7% has therefore been adopted as the glycaemic target for people with Type 1 diabetes. This has been reduced to 6.5% in a number of national guidelines, especially for people who have established complications.

Glycaemic targets in Type 2 diabetes

The United Kingdom Prospective Diabetes Study (UKPDS)[37] showed that an intensively treated group with Type 2 diabetes who had an average HbA_{1c} of 7% had reduced levels of diabetes complications when compared with a group receiving normal control who had an average HbA_{1c} of 7.9%. A level of HbA_{1c} of 7% has therefore been adopted as the glycaemic target for people with Type 2 diabetes. This has been reduced to 6.5% in a number of national guidelines, especially for people who have established complications.

Modification of targets

Intensive control of glycaemia is likely to result in more episodes of hypoglycaemia. Glycaemic targets therefore need to be negotiated individually, and need to be relaxed in the presence of significant co-morbidities. Tight glycaemic targets may seem to be counterproductive in some people. They may feel that achieving a glycaemic target of 6.5% is impossible and therefore there is no point in trying to improve their blood glucose control at all. It is vital to understand that any reduction in HbA_{1c} towards that goal is beneficial in reducing adverse outcomes. Thus lowering HbA_{1c} from 10.5% to 9% is worthwhile and will reduce adverse outcomes.[38]

Oral antihyperglycaemic agents

The results of major prospective clinical trials have emphasized the importance of achieving target glucose values. These targets are often identified by a HbA_{1c} target value established from clinical trial and epidemiologic data. As more clinical research results become available, the actual value of the glycaemic target continues to fall. The HbA_{1c} goal has been identified as a value <7%, but newer guidelines are emphasizing that the goal should be between 6 and 6.5%. It is obvious that diet and exercise will not be sufficient to achieve these targets in the majority of Type 2 diabetic patients.

A clear understanding of the pathophysiology of Type 2 diabetes is essential in planning the ideal drug therapy for the person with Type 2 diabetes. As discussed in the previous section, there are two key abnormalities: insufficient insulin secretion and increased insulin resistance. Both abnormalities play a key role in contributing to hyperglycaemia.[39]

In the person without diabetes, insulin will be secreted in two phases. There will be an initial early phase followed by a more prolonged secretion phase associated with on-going hyperglycaemia. Early phase insulin secretion plays a major role in controlling postprandial hyperglycaemia. Postprandial hyperglycaemia may play a role in the development of coronary heart disease.[40,41]

In the person with Type 2 diabetes, early phase insulin secretion is lost and the second phase may be increased and prolonged. Within 3 years of the diagnosis of Type 2 diabetes, a relative insufficiency of insulin secretion will be present, leading to increasing hyperglycaemia.

Insulin resistance can be identified when there is a failure of insulin action to carry out normal metabolic activities. Virtually all obese Type 2 diabetic patients will exhibit insulin resistance. The effects of insulin resistance are widespread and will affect multiple peripheral target tissues including fat, muscle and hepatic tissues. Insulin resistance is closely associated with the metabolic syndrome, which includes obesity, carbohydrate intolerance, hypertension and dyslipidaemia. The metabolic syndrome and insulin resistance are also strongly implicated in the development of coronary heart disease.

Drug therapies

Treatment regimens must take into account both pathophysiologic abnormalities. There is now a wide range of drugs available to treat the person with diabetes and achieve important target glucose levels (Table 7). As with the use of

Table 7. Current Type 2 oral antihyperglycaemic agents

Insulin secretagogues
Sulphonylureas
- chlorpropamide
- glibenclamide (glyburide)
- gliclazide
- glimepiride
- glipizide
- gliquidone
- tolbutamide

Meglitinides
- repaglinide

Amino acid derivatives
- nateglinide

Biguanide – decreased hepatic glucose output
- metformin

Thiazolidinediones – insulin sensitizers
- rosiglitazone
- pioglitazone

Alpha glucosidase inhibitor
- acarbose

insulin, planning an individual treatment programme will frequently produce better results than a "standard" therapeutic regimen.

Metformin

Metformin is a biguanide, which will lower blood glucose mainly through the action of reducing excessive hepatic glucose production. It is an excellent first-line drug, as it does not cause hypoglycaemia and many patients may in fact lose weight while taking the drug. The main side effects include nausea and gastrointestinal disturbances. By commencing the drug at a lower dose and titrating up slowly, these side effects can be minimized. The drug is contraindicated in patients who have kidney, heart and/or liver failure because of the slight risk of developing lactic acidosis. To help avoid gastrointestinal side effects, the drug should be commenced slowly, with 500 mg taken with supper for 3 to 4 days, and provided there are no side effects, the dose can be slowly titrated up to a maximum of 1500-2500 mg per day. If possible, at least one dose should be given at bedtime as there may be an increased benefit in terms of reducing hepatic glucose output during the night. The drug can also be given twice a day, at a dose of 850 mg.

Thiazolidinediones (TZDs)

There are two thiazolidinediones available – rosiglitazone and pioglitazone. Both of these drugs can be considered as insulin-sensitizing agents. There is increasing interest in the TZD class because it appears to provide therapeutic benefits in treating the abnormalities of the metabolic syndrome – hypertension, dyslipidaemia and hyperglycaemia. When given as monotherapy, the TZDs do not induce hypoglycaemia.[42] Recent clinical trials have suggested that the TZDs may help prevent the decline in beta-cell function that is present in Type 2 diabetes and may delay or prevent the onset of Type 2 diabetes.[43] They can be used as first-line monotherapy agents or in combination with metformin and the insulin-stimulating drugs. The TZDs have also been used as part of third-line treatment regimens when insulin-stimulating drugs, metformin and the TZDs are combined.

A small weight gain of approximately 2–4 kg is common with the use of these drugs and in a small percentage of patients, fluid retention can be an issue. Thus, these drugs should not be used in those patients with significant heart failure. TZDs are not contraindicated in patients who have had a previous myocardial infarction but whom continue to have good cardiac function.

The drug should be commenced at a starting dose of 4 mg rosiglitazone or 15 mg pioglitazone and the dose can be titrated upwards to achieve glucose targets. It is important to note that the TZD drugs can take up to 12 weeks to demonstrate their full glucose-lowering effect and thus dose changes should be made at three monthly intervals.

Fast-acting insulin secretagogues

Like sulphonylureas, nateglinide and repaglinide act through blocking potassium channels in the beta-cells. In contrast to many sulphonylureas, they have a much shorter time action and may in fact help restore first-phase insulin secretion. Thus, they are effective in lowering postprandial glucose. Because of their faster action, they tend to produce less hypoglycaemia, particularly in the first 6 months after the initiation of therapy when the risk of hypoglycaemia is highest. These drugs are usually given prior to each meal, but because of their short time action, the drug does not need to be taken if a meal is missed. This can be of particular advantage in some groups, such as older diabetic patients, who may miss lunch or other meals and thus be at increased risk of hypoglycaemia. These drugs can be started at a low dose and titrated slowly upwards to achieve target glucose values at the pre- and postprandial time periods. The major side effect is the risk of hypoglycaemia.

Slow-release insulin secretagogues

Both glimepiride and modified-release gliclazide are sulphonylurea drugs that have the capability of increasing first-phase insulin secretion and thus are good agents for controlling postprandial glucose. They are slow-release formulations, which can provide better 24-hour coverage with less hypoglycaemia

and less weight gain.[44,45] Gliclazide-MR can be commenced at
a dose of 30 mg and titrated up to 120 mg per day. Gliclazide
is also available in a multi-dose format with the initial dose
being 80mg twice daily, increasing to 160 mg twice daily as
required. Glimepiride can be commenced at a dose of 1 mg
titrating to a maximum dose of 8 mg. The major side effect is
hypoglycaemia, but with careful titration the risk is decreased.

Alpha-glucosidase inhibitors
After the ingestion of complex sugars, acarbose will delay the
conversion to the more easily absorbed simple sugars. Thus,
the most pronounced effect of acarbose is to reduce postprandial
hyperglycaemia by delaying the absorption of carbohydrates.
The lowering of postprandial glucose also leads to a significant
fall in HbA_{1c}.[46] Some long-term clinical trials have suggested
that there may be a cardiac benefit from the use of acarbose in
patients by lowering the excessive postprandial glucose rise.

The major side effect of acarbose is a significant incidence
of flatulence and diarrhoea. By introducing the drug very slowly
over a number of weeks or even months, some of these
gastrointestinal effects can be reduced or avoided.

Acarbose is ideally commenced at a low dose of 25 mg
before each meal and slowly titrated to a dose of 50-100 mg
before each meal, provided the patient does not experience
undue gastrointestinal side effects. The drug should be taken
with the first bite of the meal.

Sulphonylureas
The second-generation sulphonylureas are now most
commonly used. Glibenclamide (glyburide) is a potent
stimulator of insulin secretion. The major glucose-lowering
effect is often not experienced until 2 hours after ingestion. It
is not an ideal drug for controlling postprandial
hyperglycaemia. In addition, its duration of action can be as
long as 6–24 hours and can precipitate hypoglycaemia many
hours after the meal. In elderly patients taking sulphonylureas,
hypoglycaemia can be a major problem, particularly in those
with varying food intake.

Glibenclamide can be commenced at a dose of 2.5–5 mg before breakfast and increased to a maximum of 15 mg daily before breakfast. Glibenclamide is also given as a twice daily dose, once before breakfast and again before the evening meal. The dose is then slowly titrated to a maximum of 10 mg twice daily.

Commencing treatment

Whenever a new therapy is introduced, it must be reassessed on a regular basis, generally within 2 to 3 months of initiating the therapy. While diet and exercise remain an essential

Table 8. Clinical approach to treatment of Type 2 diabetes with oral antihyperglycaemic agents

Clinical approach

1. All of the antihyperglycaemic drugs can be considered as first-line drug therapies, but metformin is preferred in the obese patient
2. If after 3 months of any therapy, the target HbA_{1c} has not been reached, a second drug should be added in combination – combinations include metformin and a TZD, metformin and a fast-acting insulin secreting drug (repaglinide or nateglinide) or sulphonylurea (gliclazide or glimepiride); or metformin and acarbose

Rules for the clinician

1. Ensure that glucose targets are reached within 6-12 months of commencing therapy
2. Early and aggressive therapy is required with additional drug therapies being added if glucose targets are not reached within 3 months of initiating a therapy
3. Combination drug therapies will likely be necessary to achieve glucose targets and should be utilized early in the treatment regimen
4. Postprandial glucose targets should be achieved
5. Insulin resistance treated
6. New drugs should be added, rather than substituted, in ongoing drug therapy

component of management, this intervention alone will not prevent the long-term deterioration of glucose control. If the target HbA_{1c} has not been reached within 3 months of commencing a lifestyle program, drug therapy should be initiated (Table 8).

As discussed above, there are now a large number of potential drugs available for both first-line and combination therapy. Each of the drugs reviewed above can be considered as first-line therapy. There should be no longer than a 3 month trial of monotherapy, diet and exercise, and then if glucose targets have not been achieved, the second drug should be added in combination. If the target HbA_{1c} has not been reached within 3 months of commencing combination therapy, then triple drug therapy can be considered. It is very likely, however, that if triple drug therapy is required, then there will soon be a need to add insulin to the regimen.

When considering combination drugs, it is important not to combine similar classes of drugs such as utilizing two insulin-stimulating drugs. When adding a second or third drug, it is essential to maintain the original drug at its current dose and titrate the second drug to achieve target glucose levels. It is likely that in the near future, combination therapies will be commenced when drug therapy is started, rather than using a stepwise drug approach. Combination formulations are already available in some countries utilizing a combination of metformin and rosiglitazone, and metformin and sulphonylureas. These single tablet combination drugs could also help decrease the burden to the patient of taking multiple drug therapy while at the same time providing earlier and more effective treatment.

Insulin

The need to commence insulin is an issue that gives concern both to the healthcare provider, as well as to the patient. There are anxieties on the part of the prescribing physician as to whether insulin is truly required, what type of insulin should be used, what insulin regimen would best achieve the target results and whether the patient will accept a recommendation to commence insulin. For the patient, there are the concerns related to the very thought of requiring injections on a daily basis. And yet, insulin is essential for life in the Type 1 diabetic and is frequently needed in the Type 2 diabetic to obtain defined glucose targets.

There are many myths and misconceptions related to insulin therapy. Negative attitudes have been built up in the past, often related to stories of other insulin users who have had difficulties with insulin management. Each of these issues needs to be addressed and overcome (Table 9). Some of these issues include:

- If a person has been on insulin for a long time, there is no need to make any changes to an established insulin regimen.
- Yet, better understanding of the physiology of insulin action, new insulins, and taking the time to explore the patient's personal environment, can all lead to increased flexibility of lifestyle and improved glucose control.

Table 9. Excuses for not starting insulin

- patient has been on oral drugs for a long time – no need to change
- starting insulin suggests to the patient that they have reached an end-stage of their diabetes
- insulin therapy represents failure
- insulin therapy is a form of punishment for failing to achieve glucose goals
- 'benign neglect' – the healthcare professional decides it would be difficult or inconvenient for the patient

- For some patients, the decision to start insulin represents "a final stage" of their diabetes.
- This attitude is often conveyed by the healthcare professional who prescribes insulin only as a last resort in an attempt to get good glucose control. The patient comes to think of themself as a failure, and that insulin is being used as a form of punishment.
- "Benign neglect" – a situation where the healthcare professional decides what the patient might really like.
- For example, in the patient who should have been placed on multiple injections of insulin, the healthcare professional may decide that this is too much of a bother to the patient and places them only on one or two daily injections, or perhaps, a simplified insulin regimen. The patient is never actually consulted as to what their personal wishes may be in trying to achieve the targets of good glucose control.

Who needs insulin?

Obviously the Type 1 diabetic who lacks any insulin, and is c-peptide negative, will require insulin to live. In the Type 2 patient there are multiple situations where insulin administration is required. These include the patient who is failing on oral agents or is intolerant of oral agents; the patient who has significant renal or liver disease and cannot take oral antihyperglycaemic agents; gestational diabetes; and the Type 2 diabetic patient undergoing surgery (Table 10).

Table 10. Patients requiring insulin

- Type 1 diabetic with absolute insulin deficiency
- Type 2 diabetes:
  - failing on oral antihyperglycaemic agents
  - intolerant of oral agents
  - women planning a pregnancy
  - gestational diabetes
  - presence of significant renal or hepatic disease
  - glucose control during surgery

Insulin physiology and structure

In the non-diabetic individual, a basal level of insulin is secreted by the pancreatic beta-cell over a 24-hour period. Boluses of insulin are released in response to such stimuli as food, stress, and infection. The goal, when administering exogenous insulin, is to replicate this basal-bolus secretion of insulin.

Insulin consists of two amino-acid chains linked by disulphide bonds. In the pancreatic beta-cell, these two chains are linked by a connecting peptide, c-peptide, and the whole molecule is known as proinsulin. Just prior to release from the beta-cell, the c-peptide is cleaved from the insulin molecule and both insulin and c-peptide are released into circulation. Thus, the measurement of c-peptide in the serum is an excellent indicator of endogenous insulin secretion.

Human insulin molecules tend to bond together. Initially two insulin molecules will bind to form a dimer and then three dimers will join together to form a hexamer providing six molecules of insulin bound together.

This common association leads to a change of insulin activity when administering exogenous insulin. After injection, the hexamer molecules must disassociate into individual molecules to allow absorption from the subcutaneous injection

Figure 3. The structure of insulin from injection site to entry into the bloodstream

Reproduced with permission from Pickup J, Williams G. Textbook of diabetes Vol 1. Oxford: Blackwell Publishing, 1991;375.

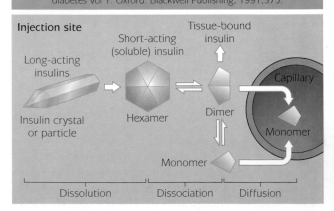

site (Figure 3). This disassociation process may take several hours. If the insulin has been administered immediately prior to a meal this will inevitably lead to a hyperglycaemic period immediately after the meal followed by increased risk of hypoglycaemia several hours after the food absorption has taken place.

By altering the structure of human insulin and creating insulin analogues, the self-association of insulin molecules has been reduced, producing monomer insulin molecules that are easily and quickly absorbed.

Exogenous insulin formulations can be classified by their time action into three groups: rapid, intermediate, and long-acting insulins. Highly purified human insulins are now produced by genetic engineering, and there is little need for the use of the older form of animal insulin. Genetic manipulation of the insulin molecule has produced analogues that more closely mimic the physiologic action of endogenous human insulin.

Analogue fast-acting insulins

The absorption of the analogue insulins differs considerably from that of soluble insulin (human regular insulin). Absorption of the analogue insulins commences within 10 minutes of injection, with peak insulin levels being reached approximately 1 hour later, compared with approximately 2 hours after injection for soluble insulin. The peak action of the analogue insulins is observed between 1 and 2 hours after injection. In contrast, the peak action of soluble insulin can be much longer, lasting 6 to 8 hours after injection. Because of the fast action of the analogues, postprandial glucose levels are far better controlled compared with soluble insulin, and the risk of hypoglycaemia is considerably reduced, particularly at night. The rapid action of the analogue insulin provides much greater flexibility in terms of the actual timing and size of the meal. In addition, some patients may have difficulty in actually determining how much they will eat at any particular time when they sit down to a meal. The fast-acting analogues can be taken during or immediately after a meal. This is of considerable benefit to patients, such as the pregnant diabetic, who may have anticipated a certain sized meal, has taken a dose of insulin, but then finds she is unable to complete all of the food. By taking the insulin during or at the end of the meal, the dose can be titrated precisely to the quantity of food that has been eaten.

Exercise will often precipitate hypoglycaemia and the dose of the analogue can be reduced if exercise takes place just after the meal. With the use of the analogues, additional snacks between meals are not required, but if a large snack is taken, for example, in excess of 15 g of carbohydrate, then additional doses of analogue can be taken to maintain euglycaemia.

The benefits of the fast-acting insulin analogues are summarized in Table 11.

Insulin lispro

Insulin lispro is formed by reversing two amino acids, proline and lysine, on the B-chain of the soluble insulin molecule. This structural change leads to a decrease in the association of the insulin dimers. By providing more rapid absorption, the physiologic profile of the insulin closely mimics endogenous human insulin.

Insulin aspart

This insulin analogue is formed when the amino acid proline is replaced by aspartic acid. This structural change again, decreases the self-association of the insulin molecules leading to more rapid absorption and action.

Table 11. Benefits of fast-acting insulin analogues

- provide insulin action closer to endogenous human insulin
- provide increased flexibility and convenience
- improve postprandial blood glucose levels
- less hypoglycaemia, particularly at night
- permit greater variability in eating and exercise

Soluble insulin (human regular insulin)

Soluble insulin was initially called a fast-acting insulin but in reality it behaves more like an intermediate-acting insulin. The insulin profile is quite different from normal endogenous physiologic insulin release. Following injection of exogenous soluble insulin there is a slow disassociation of the hexamer insulin molecules resulting in a delay of insulin absorption. After injection, peak insulin levels may not be reached until 2 hours, followed by a slow decrease. Thus, when soluble insulin has been injected, the first action of the insulin may not be seen for at least 2 hours and the peak action may last from 4 to 8 hours resulting in higher blood sugar levels after the meal and a greater risk of hypoglycaemia several hours after the meal. Thus, there is a need to ingest small snacks between meals to reduce this risk of hypoglycaemia. Not infrequently, the soluble insulin taken at suppertime, can induce hypoglycaemia in the early hours of the morning.

Ideally, soluble insulin should be injected 45–60 minutes before the beginning of each meal so that the insulin peak will coincide with the glucose rise following the meal. To reduce this inconvenience to the patient, it is generally recommended that soluble insulin be taken 30–45 minutes before the meal. Even this is often unacceptable for many patients who will take their soluble insulin immediately prior to the meal. Because of the delayed action of soluble insulin, there is reduced flexibility in altering the timing of the meal and the quantity of food that is being eaten. The key features of soluble insulin are given in Table 12.

Intermediate-acting insulin
Basal insulins

In trying to mimic normal physiologic insulin release, there is a need to establish a basal level of insulin. This is critically important in maintaining good metabolic control and additionally in achieving steady glucose values during the night. Ideally, the basal insulin should provide a steady, peakless, supply of insulin allowing addition of fast-acting insulins at appropriate times. This goal has been difficult to achieve. The

Table 12. Key features of soluble (human regular) insulin

- slow absorption rate after injection
- peak insulin levels will not be seen until 2 hours after injection
- increased insulin dose further delays the peak levels and action of the insulin
- duration of action may last 4 to 8 hours
- snacks may be required between meals
- there is increased risk of reaction 4 to 8 hours after taking the insulin
- there is poor control of postprandial hyperglycaemia
- there is increased risk of nocturnal hypoglycaemia

24-hour day can effectively be divided into two broad periods: day- and night-time. During the daytime, there will be variation of food intake and exercise. The basal insulin will provide the foundation for the fast-acting analogues or soluble insulin, which would be administered to control the intermittent glucose rise that will occur during the day. During the night, glucose levels will tend to fall until approximately 4.00 am when once again glucose production will increase and glucose levels will rise – the so-called dawn phenomenon. The basal insulin dose taken prior to bedtime, will help control glucose levels during the night and particularly in the early hours of the morning.

Isophane (NPH) insulin will generally have an onset within 2 to 4 hours after injection, reaching peak levels in the range of 4 to 12 hours. Its peak action usually occurs between 6 and 10 hours after injection, but in some patients this can be prolonged, as long as 24 hours. Insulin zinc suspension has a similar profile but in many countries its production is being discontinued.

Timing of basal insulin injections
To help control the glucose rise occurring as part of the dawn phenomenon, isophane insulin needs to be given at night.

Because of the variability of peak insulin levels from an isophane insulin injection, the timing of the injection must be carefully assessed. Ideally, the isophane insulin should be given at such a time that its main effect would be felt during the dawn phenomenon thus controlling the blood sugars immediately prior to breakfast. Not infrequently, however, isophane insulin action occurs much earlier resulting in hypoglycaemia between 1.00 and 4.00 am. The hypoglycaemia then precipitates a recovery process with increased glucose production and elevated morning glucose levels, the so-called Somogyi phenomenon. Rebound hyperglycaemia must always be suspected when the patient observes a relatively normal glucose at the time of going to sleep, but high glucose values the following morning. To help achieve the matching of insulin peak and glucose rise, isophane insulin is most frequently given at bedtime. If given at suppertime there may be an increased risk of hypoglycaemia in the early hours of the night.

Because of the relatively short action of the isophane insulin, a second dose is frequently required before breakfast to help control pre-supper blood glucose.

To try and extend the action of isophane insulin, an insulin zinc suspension has been used to provided prolonged insulin action and less of a peak effect. Insulin zinc suspension does provide an extended plasma insulin profile, but absorption is variable not only between individuals, but also within the individual diabetic patient. This results in insulin peaks occurring at different times of the day and makes it even more difficult to achieve good control of blood glucose. Some insulin companies have discontinued manufacture of insulin zinc suspension.

Long-acting insulin analogues
Neither isophane insulin with its relatively shorter action with peak levels, nor insulin zinc suspension with its erratic absorption can provide a true peakless basal insulin supply. Basal insulin with a more consistent action has now been produced by genetic engineering of the amino acid sequence of human insulin.

Insulin glargine

Human insulin is soluble in the subcutaneous tissue when the pH is 7.4. By altering the amino acid structure of human insulin the human insulin molecule can be made more soluble in acidic solutions, but once it is in the environment of a neutral pH in the subcutaneous tissue, the insulin forms micro-crystals, which take longer to absorb. In addition, the molecule can be further altered to provide a greater self-association providing further delay in absorption. The insulin glargine molecule has several amino acid changes that provide these characteristics. By delaying absorption from the injection site, insulin glargine more closely mimics the basal secretion of human insulin from the pancreatic beta-cell. Insulin glargine provides a peakless and more prolonged plasma insulin profile compared with isophane insulin. In addition, the plasma insulin profile is reproducible, both in the individual patient and in groups of diabetic patients.

In contrast to both isophane insulin and insulin zinc suspension, insulin glargine is a solution not a suspension. Prior to injection, both isophane insulin and insulin zinc suspension must be agitated to provide an even suspension for the injection. Despite this activity there is still irregularity of absorption and in addition many patients fail to agitate the vial of insulin prior to its use. Insulin glargine does not need to be re-suspended prior to injection.

Soluble insulin and fast-acting analogues can be added to isophane insulin and insulin zinc suspension, but in contrast, because of its acidic nature, other insulins cannot be added to insulin glargine.

The onset of insulin action after the injection of insulin glargine is approximately 3 to 4 hours with its effective duration being 24 hours. The insulin is ideally taken at bedtime, and because of its peakless action the dose of insulin glargine can be titrated directly against the pre-breakfast blood glucose. Thus, much lower glucose targets can be established with less risk of nocturnal hypoglycaemia. Pre-breakfast glucose values in the range of 6–7 mmol/l can be achieved with much more confidence and less hypoglycaemic events.

Table 13. Key features of insulin glargine
• steady basal insulin levels
• peakless insulin profile
• reduced nocturnal hypoglycaemia
• increased convenience
• increased flexibility of therapeutic regimens including fast-acting analogue insulins/oral agents during the daytime

By using the insulin glargine as basal insulin given at night-time, additional therapies can then be provided during the day. For the Type 1 diabetic patient, or the Type 2 diabetic patient requiring insulin, fast-acting insulin analogues or soluble insulin, can be provided during the daytime. For some Type 2 diabetic patients, the use of insulin glargine at night and the continuation of oral agents during the day can provide good glycaemic control.

A summary of the benefits of insulin glargine is provided in Table 13.

Mixed insulins

Mixed insulins are available in multiple combinations, usually combining soluble insulin with isophane insulin. The ratio is described by a series of numbers, e.g. 30/70 represents 30% soluble insulin and 70% isophane insulin (in the USA this number is reversed), or sometimes just the percentage of soluble insulin is expressed after the brand name. Different companies offer different ratios, but at present a fairly large selection is available including 10/90, 20/80, 30/70, and 50/50 insulin combinations.

These insulins are ideal for those who have a problem or some difficulty with the injection of insulin. Often they need to be given twice a day and can be given with a pen device or by syringe and needle. They are particularly useful in those who have physical or visual impairment and are most frequently used in the older patient. They are often helpful in getting a person started on insulin and once they have confidence with the insulin they can then be transferred to a more flexible regimen with insulin adjustment and thus better glucose control.

The main difficulty with these insulins is the fact that the patient actually loses flexibility and thus some control over their routine. Because the dose is fixed it is less amenable to adjustment to fit into different meal times, meal quantities, physical activity and general variations in a person's daily routine. Thus, the mixed insulin often defeats the very purpose for which the insulin is given, that is, improved glucose control.

Much of the problem with mixed insulins results from a failure to provide good education to the patient and involve them in the discussion related to target glucose values and flexibility. Hence, insulin becomes the dominant partner, with the person fitting their lifestyle around the insulin dose.

These insulins have an important role to play, but ideally should not be used in the person who has a variable lifestyle, is able to make minor adjustments to insulin, and would also like to be involved in their own personal management. Age should not be a consideration unless there are well-defined physical disabilities.

The insulin companies have now provided combinations with analogue and isophane insulin equivalents, such as biphasic insulin lispro 25 and biphasic insulin aspart 30. These do have an advantage in that they help control postprandial blood glucose better than the soluble/isophane insulin combinations.

Insulin delivery devices

Traditionally insulin has always been given by syringe injections. Different types of insulin can be combined in the same syringe and this is particularly common at breakfast time when the patient may combine intermediate-acting insulin with fast-acting insulin. When drawing two insulins, the fast-acting insulin should be drawn first followed by the intermediate-acting insulin. For many patients, however, the insulin syringe is an inconvenience. It is reasonably easy to use the syringe in the morning or at bedtime, but not infrequently, patients are

Table 14. Features of insulin pens
• provide greater flexibility
• greater portability
• allow discreet use in any environment
• helpful to elderly patients with physical or visual impairment
• help decrease the fear of injection
• provide ease of use

taking insulin throughout the day in varying situations such as their place of work, recreational venue or a restaurant. The need to draw up specific amounts of insulin and then inject the insulin can often provide inconvenience and even embarrassment.

The development of the insulin pen has completely revolutionized the manner of insulin injections (Table 14). These devices have a pen-fill ampoule of insulin inside the device and the patient merely has to attach a needle and dial the appropriate dose of insulin. It is very convenient for those who take several injections of fast-acting insulin throughout the day. The ability to carry an insulin pen inconspicuously and easily deliver the insulin, provides tremendous flexibility for all diabetic patients. For those who have a specific fear of needles, the insulin pen is less threatening and with the small, thin needle now available, the actual discomfort is minimal.

Pen use is particularly valuable to the older patient, who may have some physical or visual impairment. The insulin pen provides an easy mechanism to count the number of units being dialed without actually having to see the numbers on the display panel. The increased portability – no syringes or bottles of insulin – allows the patient to take insulin whenever and wherever they wish.

Variability of insulin action

Insulin action can vary between different diabetic patients but also within individuals. It is important to establish what the pattern of insulin action is with each individual patient and

Table 15. Variability of insulin action

- variability exists between different patients
- variability exists within individual patients
- insulin injection sites need to be rotated
- using the abdomen as an injection site provides more even, predictable absorption rates
- absorption of insulin is increased from an exercising limb
- a warm environment – hot baths/showers/saunas will lead to increased absorption rates
- the depth of the insulin injection will alter absorption rates
- the size of the insulin needle alters absorption rates
- the time the insulin needle is within the subcutaneous tissue will alter absorption rates

watch for potential changes. There are a number of situations that can cause a variation in insulin action (Table 15).

The site of injection is important. The patient can choose to rotate injection sites around a specific area or rotate throughout many body areas. Injection in the abdomen generally provides a more even and predictable absorption rate and is preferred by most diabetic patients. Insulin can be injected anywhere on the body, but scar tissue or thickened skin, can alter the absorption rate. If insulin is injected into an exercising limb, absorption rates can be increased, thus precipitating a faster action of the insulin and potential hypoglycaemia. Similar changes can be expected with the use of hot baths/showers/saunas.

The depth of injection can also alter absorption rates. The type of needle may also influence absorption rates when the short, thin needles are used in obese patients. It is advisable to leave the needle in the tissue for 5–10 seconds after injection to reduce leakage.

Initiating insulin

Successfully initiating insulin requires adherence to two important concepts – the development of a flexible insulin regimen, and a regimen that has been individualized to the specific patient. It is important that the insulin regimen is designed to fit into the patient's personal life and activities, rather than imposing a system whereby the patient struggles to manage their meals, physical activities, and social life in the framework of a rigid insulin administration programme. While there are established guidelines as to how insulin can be administered, and there is considerable knowledge as to the time action and dynamics of specific insulins, there are in fact no set rules. The goal is to mimic as closely and as safely as possible the daily release of insulin that might be seen in a non-diabetic patient in response to activities such as eating, exercise, stress, and relaxation.

It is important to establish glycaemic goals that are practical and attainable taking into account the patients age, dexterity, vision, activities and variability of their personal lifestyle.

As insulin is commenced, it must be expected that there will be extensive metabolic effects. Insulin is the most powerful agent to lower glucose, but in addition, will decrease fat cell catabolism, decrease excess hepatic glucose production, and provide storage of food. The main side effect of the use of insulin is hypoglycaemia and this is extensively reviewed in Section: Hypoglycaemia (pages 84–93). In addition, as insulin is commenced, the patient may experience considerable weight gain and will need dietary guidance.

It is important to realize that the goal of initiating insulin therapy is to control hyperglycaemia and protect the patient from development of long-term vascular complications. Ideally, the administered insulin should mimic the natural production of endogenous insulin and as new insulins are developed, this goal is becoming more attainable. In addition, to achieve the important goal of flexibility and reaching glucose targets in a safe manner, it is apparent that multiple injections of insulin each day will be required.

Factors affecting an insulin dose

There is no "correct" insulin dose – it must be adapted to each person and their personal lifestyle. Before commencing insulin therapy, it is valuable to spend some time talking to the patient about their daily routine. By asking several key questions, it becomes easier to define the type of insulin to be used and when it should be given. There are several areas of the patient's personal history that should be explored and these are illustrated in Table 16. Within the contexts of such a short conversation, lies the "design" of an individualized insulin regimen.

Choice of insulins

The goal in using insulin is to achieve glucose control with a flexible, safe insulin regimen. This aim is best achieved by using a combination of insulins, which will provide a basal level of insulin throughout a 24-hour period, as well as bolus injections before meal times.

The basal insulin levels can be achieved with isophane insulin given at bedtime and usually before breakfast. The bolus injection is provided by using a fast-acting insulin before breakfast and supper. For many, the addition of a bolus dose prior to lunch provides even greater flexibility and improved glucose control.

Bedtime insulin

Insulin given before going to bed is designed to maintain a steady glucose level overnight. The goal is to achieve approximately the same glucose levels at bedtime and again the following morning. For example, if the bedtime glucose is in the range of 10 mmol/l, then the pre-breakfast glucose level should be in the range of 9–11 mmol/l. Similarly if the bedtime glucose is 7 mmol/l the pre-breakfast blood sugar the next morning should be in the range of 6–8 mmol/l. If the bedtime glucose is elevated, it is not the role of the night-time insulin to decrease the value overnight. This merely increases the risk of nocturnal hypoglycaemia. More logically, the reason for the elevated bedtime glucose value should be identified and the appropriate corrections made for subsequent evenings. The use of bedtime bolus fast-acting insulin should be avoided if possible, as the risk of nocturnal hypoglycaemia is once again increased. In the presence of significant bedtime

Table 16. Factors affecting an insulin dose

Food intake

- what are your general eating habits
  - do you eat at home?
  - at work?
  - in restaurants?

- how do you distribute your daily calories
  - do you snack throughout the day?
  - eat regular meals?
  - are some meals larger than others are – for example is supper the largest meal?
  - do you miss meals?
  - what can cause a change in your eating habits – work, illness
  - do you regularly take a snack at bedtime?
  - what can cause a change in food intake – work, home, activities, exercise

(don't forget the home-maker who may have the most variable daily routine of all patients)

Activities

- do you exercise on a regular basis
  - most days?

- at specific times
  - the extent of the exercise?
  - the type of exercise?

Work routines

- do you work at home?
- do you have a specific place of work?
- does your work routine vary on a daily basis?
- is it physical or sedentary?
- do you have shift work hours?

Specific issues

- during your daily routine how many unexpected or unpredictable events can occur?
- do you get frequent infections?
- what events appear to cause a major disturbance in your blood glucose control?
- do you have any physical disabilities that might prevent you giving an insulin injection

hyperglycaemia a small bolus dose can be taken with the major glucose correction taking place prior to breakfast the next day. Once the ideal basal bedtime insulin dose has been established, it rarely needs major adjustments.

The pre-breakfast basal isophane insulin dose helps to control the post-lunch and pre-supper glucose levels with a diminished effect after supper. Generally, more insulin will be required in the morning compared with the bedtime dose.

It is likely that the long-acting analogue insulins, such as glargine, will be used preferentially as the bedtime basal insulin. The use of the long-acting insulin glargine alters the need for a pre-breakfast isophane insulin basal dose. Because of the 20–24 hour action of insulin glargine, it can be given at bedtime and the dose titrated to achieve a pre-breakfast glucose level in the range of 6–7 mmol/l. The dose of insulin glargine needs to be adjusted if there is evidence of nocturnal hypoglycaemia.

Insulin glargine can be used in combination with the daytime use of oral agents or analogue insulins.

Daytime insulin
The bolus fast-acting insulin becomes the "fine-adjuster" of the daytime period. Ideally, analogue fast-acting insulins should be used to gain the greatest flexibility for the patient, with better control of the postprandial glucose and decreased risk of hypoglycaemia. The actual dose of the analogue insulin can be calculated according to the size and content of the specific meal and the potential physical activities after the meal. Many patients employ the concept of carbohydrate counting to establish the ideal analogue dose. The analogue insulin can be given before breakfast, lunch, or supper depending on the wishes of the specific patient. If a lunchtime dose is employed, the morning basal isophane insulin will probably need to be decreased by 20–30%.

When titrating analogue insulins, keep it logical, and keep it simple.

The peak effect of the analogue insulin occurs 2 hours after the injection and thus the analogue insulin dose can be titrated based on the glucose level 2 hours post-injection. This of course corresponds with the key postprandial period. A safe glucose goal to seek would be a value of 8–10 mmol/l either immediately prior to the next meal or 2 hours after the meal. It is important to establish a simple regimen, which includes glucose monitoring and insulin adjustment to achieve these goals. There is little need for very complex regimens and in fact, many of these regimens do not succeed because of their complexity.

Rather than impose a rigid glucose monitoring schedule upon the patient, ask the patient how many glucose tests a week they are prepared to do, then utilize this number to ensure tests are conducted at key times to permit appropriate insulin adjustment. Many patients like the concept of glucose-testing patterning (Table 17). This allows for a steady progression of insulin adjustment over key time periods. A typical example of glucose-testing patterning would be asking the patient to measure for a 2-week period, the pre-breakfast and 2-hour post-breakfast glucose. It is not essential for it to be done every day, but within 2 weeks, the patient will have experienced most of the variable aspects of their personal lives, e.g. differing morning blood glucoses, differing breakfast quantities, and differing activities after the meal. With the goal being 8–10 mmol/l in the 2-hour postprandial period, the patient can then make appropriate adjustments to the analogue insulin dose to achieve these goals and also learn the ideal dose of the analogue insulin for most eventualities. Once the pre-breakfast analogue dose has been established, the same process can be repeated at lunchtime and then at supper.

Table 17. Glucose-testing patterning

- glucose-testing before, and 2 hours after a meal
- the correct insulin dose is established as part of the patient's daily routine
- develops flexibility
- encourages active participation by the patient
- establishes the patient as the dominant person in deciding the appropriate insulin dose

Managing the Type 1 diabetes patient with insulin

For the Type 1 diabetes patient, insulin is essential and the basal-bolus concept is ideal to permit the patient to achieve good glucose target levels and at the same time maintain a satisfactory quality of life. It is important not to allow the concept of glucose monitoring and insulin adjustment to dominate their daily routine.

Obviously, there are multiple insulin regimens that will suit a specific patient, but the concept of a basal insulin dose with multiple injections of short-acting insulins throughout the day will provide the best opportunity to achieve target glucose values (Table 18). Ideally the Type 1 diabetes patient should be commenced on a programme of at least three insulin injections a day. An isophane insulin dose can be given at bedtime and again at breakfast, with an analogue insulin taken at breakfast, lunch, and supper. Insulin glargine can be substituted for bedtime isophane insulin and a morning isophane insulin dose is then not required.

There is no precise insulin dose when commencing insulin in a new Type 1 diabetes patient. At the time of diagnosis, the patient may in fact be insulin resistant and higher doses will be required as insulin is initiated.

Table 18. Examples of insulin regimens for Type 1 diabetes

Insulin type	Breakfast	Lunch	Supper	Bedtime
Example 1				
Isophane insulin	X			X
Regular/analogue	X		X	
Example 2				
Isophane insulin	X			X
Regular/analogue	X	X	X	
Example 3				
Isophane/glargine				X
Regular/analogue	X	X	X	

Some physicians, when initiating insulin, prefer to use a basic formula to help choose the correct dose of insulin. Approximately one half to two thirds of the total daily insulin is provided by the basal insulin dose and the remainder by the short-acting insulin. The actual dose of insulin can be estimated by calculating the following formula:

$$body\ weight\ in\ kg \times 0.6$$

Thus, for the 70 kg patient, the initial insulin dose would be $70 \times 0.6 = 42$ units per day. This total dose would then be divided into basal insulin and fast-acting insulin doses. This dose must be adjusted for variations in the patient's food intake and exercise routine. It is preferable to start with a lower insulin dose and then increase as required, rather than making an error in providing too much insulin at the beginning of the therapy and inducing hypoglycaemia.

Honeymoon period

Shortly after commencing insulin, the patient may enter a phase known as the honeymoon period when endogenous insulin secretion once again becomes more effective. Insulin requirements may decrease and glucose levels may become more stable. It is important to continue regular glucose monitoring and not to stop insulin. The honeymoon phase can persist for many months and even up to 1 year but, inevitably, the endogenous insulin secretion will cease and the patient will be totally dependent on exogenous insulin.

Managing the Type 2 diabetes patient with insulin

In reality the goal is the same – good glucose control while at the same time trying to minimize the impact of diabetes management on the person's daily routine. For many Type 2 diabetes patients, insulin will be the key to achieving better glucose control and the lowering of glucose targets, it is expected that many Type 2 diabetes patients will require insulin to achieve these targets. It is important to remember that diet and exercise remain the cornerstone of management in all diabetes patients.

Basal insulin may often be all that is required to achieve good glucose control. Either isophane insulin or insulin glargine can be given at bedtime to achieve the same targets, as described above. Many may be able to maintain daily oral therapies to achieve target glucose values. If these glucose values are not achieved, however, insulin will also be required during the day. Again there are multiple insulin regimens that might suit any specific patient (Table 19).

The bedtime basal isophane insulin, as well as breakfast isophane insulin can be given and tablets maintained during the day. If available, insulin glargine can be given at bedtime with oral agents taken during the day. The use of metformin in combination with insulin can often be beneficial in helping to decrease the weight gain associated with insulin use and to provide some increased sensitivity to the insulin action. Insulin-sensitizing agents (TZDs) have also been used with insulin to help reduce the necessity of large insulin doses, but in some people, this will lead to an increased risk of oedema, and the attendant risk of heart failure means this combination must be used with caution. Indeed, the combination of insulin and a

Table 19. Examples of insulin regimens for Type 2 diabetes

Insulin type	Breakfast	Lunch	Supper	Bedtime
Example 1				
Isophane insulin	X			X
Regular/analogue	X		X	
Example 2				
Isophane insulin	X			X
Regular/analogue	X	X	X	
Example 3				
Isophane/glargine				X
Regular/analogue	X	X	X	
Example 4				
Glargine/isophane				X
Oral agents	X	X	X	

TZD is currently contraindicated in the UK and Europe. If the use of basal insulins and oral agents do not achieve defined glucose targets, there will be a need for basal-bolus regimens using basal insulins at night and in the morning, and analogue or soluble insulins during the day (Tables 20 and 21).

Storage of insulin

Prior to use, insulin should be stored in the refrigerator. As injecting cold insulin can be painful, an opened insulin container can be safely kept at room temperature for approximately 1 month. In those countries where there may be extremes of temperature, insulin can be safely transported inside a thermos flask.

Pump therapy

The introduction of the sophisticated, programmable insulin pump has provided another avenue of insulin injection for the highly motivated patient. The insulin pump works on the principle of continuous insulin infusion where the basal insulin can be programmed for different times of the day. In addition,

Table 20. Mixing insulins

- after mixing, use soon
- commercially prepared insulins can be stored for long periods of time
- mixing cannot be done with insulin glargine
- draw rapid insulins first

Table 21. Insulin adjustment

- if there is need to decrease insulin – do it
- if a possible need to increase insulin – think about it
- use glucose patterning to establish insulin dosages
- achieve a steady glucose level between bedtime and breakfast using basal insulins
- achieve a postprandial glucose in the range of 8-10 mmol/l

bolus insulin doses can be provided at any time of the day to fit into a variable work schedule and meal routine. The patient seeking to use pump therapy should be experienced in insulin use and prepared to monitor blood glucose levels multiple times throughout the day. Ideally, a person should be commenced on pump therapy within a well-established pump-education programme supervised by a physician experienced in pump therapy.

Future developments

Considerable research is now taking place in the methods of insulin delivery. Inhaled insulin has proven to be effective and major trials are now underway to assess its safety. An oral spray insulin has also been developed and extensive studies are evaluating its efficacy and safety. Other methods of insulin delivery such as a skin patch and oral tablets are also being investigated.

Helpful hints

1. Ensure that the patient understands the actions of the insulin so that they too can help in the process of insulin adjustment
2. Set attainable and safe glucose targets
3. Emphasize that insulin can provide improved glucose control within a variable lifestyle
4. Introduce the patient to the insulin pen concept
5. Emphasize that the patient is in charge of the insulin regimen not the healthcare professional

Microvascular complications

Diabetic eye disease

Diabetes accelerates cataract formation, but has its main damaging effects on the retinal blood vessels, causing diabetic retinopathy. This is the most common cause of blindness in the working population of the Western world.

The prevalence of retinopathy increases with duration of diabetes and worsening of glycaemic control. In one study of people with Type 2 diabetes, 20% had evidence of retinopathy within 2 years of diagnosis and 60% within 15 years of diagnosis.[47]

Retinopathy progression

Some of the earliest subclinical abnormalities of the retinal blood vessels include thickening of the basement membrane, loss of pericyte cells (contractile cells that alter vessel calibre and flow), increased retinal blood flow and capillary permeability.

Microaneurysms are usually the first clinical signs of retinal blood vessel damage. Hard exudates are flakes of plasma protein and lipid that have leaked from retinal blood vessels. They can affect vision if they occur in the macula.

Cotton wool spots are whitish elevations of the nerve fibre layer. Progression from background retinopathy to preproliferative is due to worsening retinal ischaemia. IRMAs, abnormally branched vessels in the retina, occur as the ischaemic retina attempts to revascularize.

Proliferative retinopathy is characterized by the formation of many more abnormal new blood vessels, stimulated by the release of growth factors from the ischaemic retina.

Advanced diabetic eye disease occurs when further vitreous contraction pulls on strong fibrous adhesions connecting the retina and vitreous, and produces retinal detachment and vitreous haemorrhage.

Table 22. Classification of retinopathy

	Features	Symptoms
Grade 1.	*Background*	
	microaneurysms	none
	venous dilatation	
	scattered exudates	
	dot & blot haemorrhages	
Grade 2.	*Preproliferative*	
	cotton wool spots	none
	multiple haemorrhages	
	intraretinal microvascular abnormalities (IRMA)	
	venous beading, looping and duplication	
Grade 3.	*Proliferative*	
	new vessels on disc and elsewhere	none if uncomplicated but haemorrhage
	fibrous proliferation on disc and elsewhere	may give visual loss
	preretinal and vitreous haemorrhages	
Grade 4.	*Advanced diabetic eye disease*	
	retinal detachment and tears	visual loss or blindness
	extensive fibrovascular proliferation	
	vitreous haemorrhage	
	neovascular glaucoma	
Grade 5.	*Maculopathy*	
	macular oedema	central visual loss
	ischaemic maculopathy	

Screening for diabetic eye disease

The key issue is to identify those people with sight-threatening retinopathy who will benefit from preventive treatment to prevent visual loss. These individuals may well be asymptomatic.

In the UK it is recommended that people with Type 2 diabetes need screening once the diagnosis is made and annually thereafter.[48] A number of people (estimations vary between 20 and 40%) will have evidence of retinopathy at diagnosis. This indicates that they may well have had Type 2 diabetes for a number of years before diagnosis.

Screening used to be based on observing the retina through a dilated pupil using an ophthalmoscope (direct ophthalmoscopy). However, significant numbers of people with sight-threatening retinopathy may be missed using this technique, even when it is carried out by ophthalmologists. It is therefore being replaced in many countries by either digital retinal photography or observing the retina using a slit lamp and Volk lens (indirect ophthalmoscopy).

UK Guidelines suggest that screening should be carried out using a test that has been demonstrated to have a sensitivity of 80% or higher and a specificity of 95% or higher, and a technical failure rate of 5% or less.[48] Direct ophthalmoscopy cannot achieve these levels of sensitivity and specificity.

People with Type 1 diabetes need screening yearly from puberty onwards or after 5 years from diagnosis whichever is the shorter period.

The advantage of digital retinal photography is that it is easily audited and the digital image can be easily stored and retrieved. It may also become automated in the future as computer software is being developed to read digital photographs and screen out those that are normal.

There is some emerging evidence that "dual modality" screening, looking at the retina through a slit lamp and then taking a digital retinal photograph, may become the "gold standard" in the future.

In some countries screening by indirect ophthalmoscopy, which is usually carried out by trained optometrists, is most common, in others, screenings based on digital photography is the emerging modality of choice. In some countries both screening methods are used.

The role of the family physician is to ensure that the person with diabetes has an annual retinal screening test using the preferred local modality, and that this information is added to the patients clinical records. It is vital that any abnormalities that constitute sight-threatening retinopathy are detected and the patient referred for urgent review and laser therapy to preserve sight (Table 23).

Treatment of retinopathy
Optimize glycaemic control

Strict control of glycaemia will reduce both the incidence and progression of early retinopathy. This has been shown for people with Type 1 diabetes in the DCCT study[36] and for people with Type 2 diabetes in the UKPDS study.[37] In this latter study the strict control group maintained a 0.9% lower HbA_{1c} level than those in the conventional group and this resulted in a 25% reduction in microvascular endpoints, most marked in the need for laser photocoagulation. For every 1% reduction in HbA_{1c} there is a 37% decrease in laser treatment and a 10% reduction in cataract extraction.[38]

Table 23. Referral to an opthalmology specialist

Same day
- sudden loss of vision and retinal detachment

Within 1 week
- new vessels, preretinal or vitreous haemorrhage
- rubeosis iridis

Within 4 weeks
- unexplained drop in visual acuity, hard exudates within 1 disc diameter of fovea
- macular oedema
- pre-proliferative or severe retinopathy

Within 3–6 months
- worsening of lesions since previous screen
- scattered exudates more than 1 disc diameter from fovea

Optimize blood pressure control

In the UKPDS blood pressure study, tight control of blood pressure aiming at below 150/90 mmHg had a significant beneficial effect in reducing the incidence of retinopathy and its progression to laser photocoagulation.[49] For every 10mmHg reduction in systolic blood pressure there was an 11% reduction in the need for laser treatment. Only 10% of people with tight blood pressure control lost three lines of vision on the Snellen chart while in the less tightly controlled group 20% did so.[50]

Referral for laser photocoagulation

Laser treatment is effective in treating sight-threatening retinopathy, proliferative retinopathy and maculopathy characterized by fluid accumulation in the immediate vicinity of the fovea. The greatest effect is seen in proliferative retinopathy where, with adequate and timely treatment, useful central vision can be maintained in up to 90% of patients.[50] This is often achieved only by sacrificing peripheral vision, which in some patients means they will not fulfil the visual requirements needed to be able to continue to drive.

Many people with retinopathy have normal vision and do not know that they may be developing a potentially sight-threatening condition. Regular screening is vital to detect these changes.

Refer for eye surgery

Vitrectomy is usually successful in certain forms of advanced diabetic retinopathy: non-clearing vitreous haemorrhage, traction on the macula, and retinal detachment involving the macula. These complications can also sometimes occur in proliferative retinopathy if the condition has not been treated in good time or adequately.

Prevention of retinopathy

The results of the DCCT and UKPDS trials have shown that optimizing blood glucose control to an HbA_{1c} of 7% and optimizing blood pressure control (140/80 mmHg or below) reduces the risk of developing retinopathy.

The possibility that ACE inhibitors might limit the progression of retinopathy in normotensive people with Type 1 diabetes was suggested in one study[51] but the study group commented that further controlled trials would be needed before changes in clinical practice would be advocated.

Retinopathy screening and management summary

Actions for family physician

After diagnosis of Type 2 diabetes and at appropriate time after diagnosis of Type 1 diabetes refer for examination to detect retinopathy

if no retinopathy present

- arrange recall for annual review (ensure that it happens)

if retinopathy present

- optimize glycaemic control
- optimize blood pressure control (manage according to severity)

emergency referral to ophthalmology specialist (same day)

- sudden loss of vision
- retinal detachment

urgent referral to ophthalmology specialist (within 1 week)

- new vessels
- preretinal and/or vitreous haemorrhage
- rubeosis iridis

referral to ophthalmology specialist (within 4 weeks)

- unexplained drop in visual acuity
- hard exudates within 1 disc diameter of fovea
- macular oedema
- pre-proliferative or severe retinopathy

recall and review (every 3 – 6 months)

- worsening of lesions since previous examination
- scattered exudates more than 1 disc diameter from fovea

routine care (screen yearly)

- minimal or background retinopathy

Cataract

Is more common in people with diabetes, and the incidence is reduced where glycaemic levels are optimized.[38] Where cataract is interfering with vision or preventing assessment of the retina, cataract extraction surgery needs to be contemplated.

Nephropathy

Nephropathy is the diabetes microvascular complication that occurs in the kidney. Hypertension is a feature and can be a pre-disposing factor.

The main site of pathology is in the glomerulus where there is basement membrane thickening and expansion of the mesangium that results in a declining glomerular filtration rate. In advanced diabetic renal disease nodular glomerulosclerosis occurs (Kimmelsteil–Wilson kidney). As more damage occurs to the kidney so there is an increasing amount of protein leakage into the urine.

Natural history

There is a progression from normoalbuminuria (leakage of below 30 mg in 24 hours), through a phase of microalbuminuria (leakage of 30–300 mg in 24 hours) to dipstick positive proteinuria (more than 300 mg in 24 hours).

Once persistent dipstick positive proteinuria has developed, renal function usually declines slowly and progressively towards end-stage renal failure with the need for dialysis or renal transplantation.

About 20% of people with Type 1 diabetes have proteinuria after a disease duration of 25 years.[52] The cumulative incidence of microalbuminuria in people with Type 1 diabetes at 30 years' disease duration is approximately 40%.[52]

The prevalence of proteinuria in people with Type 2 diabetes is approximately 15%.[53] The cumulative incidence of microalbuminuria in people with Type 2 diabetes at 10 years' disease duration is approximately 20–25%.[53]

In Type 1 diabetes many people with microalbuminuria will be normotensive. In Type 2 diabetes the majority of people with microalbuminuria will have hypertension.

Microalbuminuria is a marker of endothelial dysfunction and indicates an increased risk of generalized atherosclerosis. It is associated with an increased mortality from cardiovascular disease.

Monitoring of renal function in diabetes

As part of a diabetes annual review, serum creatinine should be measured and an early morning specimen of urine dipstick-tested for proteinuria.

In those people who are negative for dipstick proteinuria a morning specimen of urine should be checked for the presence of microalbuminuria by sending the specimen for estimation of the albumin/creatinine ratio. A ratio of 2.5 mg/mmol and above in adult men and 3.5 mg/mmol or greater in women are diagnostic of microalbuminuria.

Risk factors for the development of nephropathy

Risk factors include hyperglycaemia, raised blood pressure, baseline albumin excretion, increasing age, duration of diabetes, presence of retinopathy, smoking, genetic factors, raised cholesterol and trigylceride levels, male sex, and elevated serum homocysteine levels.[31]

Prevention of nephropathy

Good glycaemic control with a target HbA_{1c} of 7% should be maintained in all people with diabetes to reduce the risk of developing nephropathy.

In the DCCT study a reduction in mean HbA_{1c} from 9% to 7% was associated with a 39% reduction in the occurrence of microalbuminuria, and a 54% reduction in the occurrence of proteinuria in people with Type 1 diabetes.[36] In the UKPDS a reduction in mean HbA_{1c} from 7.9% to 7% was associated with a risk reduction of developing microalbuminuria of 11%, and proteinuria by 3.5% in people with Type 2 diabetes.[37]

Tight blood pressure control (140/80 mmHg or less) in patients with Type 2 diabetes should be maintained to reduce the risk of developing diabetic nephropathy.

The UKPDS study in people with Type 2 diabetes showed a reduction in mean blood pressure from 154/87 mmHg in the conventional group to 144/82 mmHg in the tight control group was associated with an absolute risk reduction for developing microalbuminiuria of 8% over 6 years.[49]

More aggressive management programmes to control blood pressure in people with established nephropathy are being proposed, with levels of 135/75 mmHg or less becoming the target to aim for in these high-risk groups.

Treatment of people with Type 1 diabetes who have persistent microalbuminuria

Many will not have hypertension. There is now good evidence that treatment with an ACE inhibitor[54] or if not tolerated an angiotension II receptor antagonist can preserve renal function and decrease microalbuminuria.

Treatment of people with Type 2 diabetes who have persistent microalbuminuria

Many will have hypertension already. They may already be on an ACE inhibitor or an angiotensin II receptor antagonist to treat the hypertension. If they are not, one should be used as there is evidence in Type 2 diabetes that these agents are beneficial in preserving renal function and decreasing microalbuminuria.[55,56]

Treatment with a low protein diet

Reduction of dietary protein intake to 0.6–0.8 g/kg/day reduces the rate of glomerular filtration rate loss in people with Type 1 diabetes who have proteinuria and impaired renal function.[57] Such low protein diets need to be initiated and supervized by a dietician and renal team. There is no evidence for their use in people with Type 2 diabetes.[31]

Non-diabetic causes of renal problems

Proteinuria or renal impairment in people with Type 2 diabetes may be due to non-diabetic causes, including glomerulnephritis and pyleonephritis. Non-diabetes causes may be suspected if there is an absence of retinopathy, haematuria and rapidly progressive renal impairment, and rapid referral to a renal specialist is required.

Referral for renal replacement therapy

There is no specific evidence to advise on the correct time to refer to a renal clinic, however most renal physicians would prefer patients to be referred earlier rather than later. Some guidelines suggest referral when the serum creatinine exceeds 150 μmol/l.[31]

Renal replacement therapy consists of haemodialysis, continuous ambulatory peritoneal dialysis (CAPD) and renal transplantation. Assessment for, and initiation of, renal replacement therapy is undertaken by a specialist renal team. In many countries diabetes is one of the leading causes of renal failure, accounting for more than one in six people starting renal replacement therapy.

Nephropathy summary

Actions for family physician

- measure serum creatinine yearly
  - if over 150 μmol/l refer to specialist
- measure urine albumin:creatinine ratio
  - use a first morning sample
  - send to laboratory or use near-patient specific test

  if negative – repeat yearly

  if positive – repeat twice within 1 month

  if two out of three are positive, microalbuminuria is confirmed

Management of those who have confirmed microalbuminuria

- if retinopathy not present consider non-diabetic causes of renal disease
- consider referral to specialist
- begin therapy with ACE inhibitor or angiotensin II receptor antagonist
- maintain blood pressure below 135/75 mmHg
  - combinations of agents are likely to be needed
- optimize glycaemic control aiming for HbA$_{1c}$ below 6.5–7.5% according to the individual's target
- assess and manage cardiovascular risk factors aggressively

Diabetic neuropathy and the diabetic foot

People with diabetes may suffer from a variety of polyneuropathies and mononeuropathies. However, chronic sensorimotor neuropathy is by far the most common to occur as a microvascular complication of diabetes. A number of population and clinic-based epidemiological studies have given estimates of prevalence of 23–46%.[58]

The onset of the chronic neuropathy is gradual and insidious in many people. Clinical examination usually reveals a sensory deficit in the lower limb in a bilateral stocking distribution. Signs of motor dysfunction may be present with wasting of small muscles in the foot and absent ankle jerks.

Neuropathy symptoms

There can be a spectrum of symptoms, with a few people experiencing severe symptoms of sharp, shooting, stabbing pains with parasthesiae and hyperaesthesiae, which are often worse at night. Some people experience only an occasional mild symptom and many have no symptoms at all, and are unaware of the loss of protective pain sensation that the neuropathy has given them.

A history of typical symptoms is strongly suggestive of diabetic peripheral neuropathy, but an absence of symptoms does not exclude neuropathy. In many it can only be detected by examination.

A number of drugs including amitriptyline given at doses of 25 to 150 mg at bedtime can improve symptomatic neuropathy, but no drug presently available affects the natural history of the condition, and nerve function gradually deteriorates.[59]

Autonomic neuropathy

Sympathetic autonomic neuropathy in people with diabetes can cause a wide variety of symptoms including postural hypotension and diarrhoea. In the lower limb it can result in reduced sweating, and increased blood flow. This can cause the skin of the foot to dry and make it prone to crack, thus increasing the risk of foot infection.

Diabetic foot ulceration and amputation

Data from foot clinics suggest that up to 90% of people attending with foot ulcers have clinical evidence of neuropathy. A large multicentre study has reported a 7% annual risk of ulceration in people with diabetic neuropathy (Figure 4).[58]

The neuropathic foot does not spontaneously ulcerate. It is the combination of neuropathy with its resulting loss of protective pain sensation, plus at least one other factor, which may be extrinsic, such as ill-fitting footware, other minor trauma, scalds and heat injury, or intrinsic, such as high foot pressures and callus formation, that results in ulceration.

Screening for neuropathy in the foot

Identification of neuropathy based on insensitivity to a 10 g nylon monofilament is convenient and appears to be cost-effective.[53] The monofilament was originally developed for screening in leprosy, which causes a neuropathy similar to that seen in diabetes.

The filament is applied to at least five sites on the forefoot (but not over callus) until it buckles, which occurs at 10 g of linear pressure. The person being screened is asked to say each time they can feel it touching, if it is not detected then protective pain sensation has been lost and the foot is "at risk" of ulceration (Figure 5).

Figure 4. Foot ulcer as a consequence of diabetic neuropathy

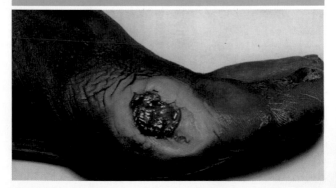

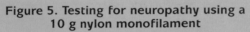

Figure 5. Testing for neuropathy using a 10 g nylon monofilament

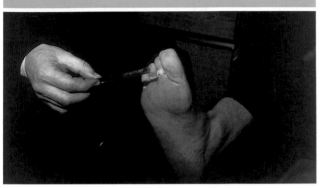

Testing with the monofilament has been shown to have excellent within and between observer reproducibility and good specificity for the detection of peripheral neuropathy.[60] In a study conducted in an outpatient clinic looking at the reproducibility of screening using a variety of methods, only the monofilament gave adequately reproducible results (over 85%) for measurements repeated after 2 weeks.

Other factors contribute to the "at risk" status of feet of people with diabetes including:

- history of previous ulceration
- presence of bone deformity and callus
- presence of ischaemia, as detected by absent foot pulses.

These risk factors can be assessed in about 90 seconds by asking people at their annual review examination to take off their shoes and socks, and then:

- asking about any history of previous ulceration
- inspecting the feet for signs of bone deformity and callus
- palpating the dorsalis pedis and posterior tibial pulses
- applying the 10 g nylon monofilament to at least five sites on each foot.

Insensitivity to the 10 g monofilament has been used to develop a simple ladder of increasing risk, with the normal foot as 0, the insensate foot as 1, the insensate and deformed foot as 2 and history of previous ulceration as 3. Such a scheme has

Diagnosis and management of foot problems summary

Responsibilities of family physician
- examine feet at diagnosis and then every year
  - examine feet to detect foot "at risk"
    by inspecting feet for bony abnormalities and callus
    palpation of pulses
    use of 10 g nylon monofilament to detect insensitivity
if any of above are abnormal foot is "at risk"
- refer for extra education and review
if all are normal
- check again at next annual review
if person newly presents with ulceration and/or cellulitis
- refer urgently to multidisciplinary footcare team

been tested in primary care in the USA where 358 people with diabetes were followed for 32 months. Forty-one people developed foot ulceration and incidence rates correlated positively with increasing risk category. All 14 amputations occurred in risk groups 2 and 3.[61]

Follow up after annual review foot "at risk" examination
If foot is normal – Give general foot care advice and a general foot care leaflet. Repeat at annual review in 1 year's time.

If foot is "at risk" – Refer to local foot "at risk" clinic where more detailed education, investigation and 3 monthly follow up can be instituted.

Referral of acute foot problems
International guidelines on the management of diabetic neuropathy advise that patients presenting acutely with ulceration, blistering, bleeding into callus, cellulitis or acute ischaemia should be referred immediately, usually on the day of presentation.[62]

This referral should be to the local multidisciplinary diabetes footcare team. This team should ideally be made up of a specialist podiatrist, diabetologist, and diabetes nurse who have immediate access to general and vascular surgery, and orthotic expertise.

Such a team can ensure that the person with an acute foot problem can quickly receive debridement and appropriate dressing of their acute lesion, antibiotics where necessary, and treatment to normalize blood glucose levels. They then need to be mobilized quickly in special footwear to ensure that pressure on the damaged area of the foot is "off loaded" and healing promoted.

A number of centres around the world have published uncontrolled studies showing reductions in amputation rates of 40% or more through screening, education and the development of such teams. One team was able to demonstrate a reduction in amputations of 40%, and healing rates of 86% for ulcers that were mainly neuropathic in aetiology. Relapse rates in those who wore special footwear were 26% compared with a rate of 83% in those who wore their own shoes.[63]

Many parts of the world do not, as yet, have such multidisciplinary footcare teams working in dedicated clinics. The podiatrist with a special interest in diabetes foot problems may be the best person to refer to in those circumstances.

Erectile dysfunction

This is the major sexual problem affecting men with diabetes. It affects over 30% of all men who have diabetes and 55% of those over 60 years of age.[64] The prevalence and impact of erectile failure in diabetes is probably underestimated because of medical and social taboos.

Its aetiology is multifactorial. The main two factors are atheroma causing reduced blood flow to the penis, and damage to the autonomic nervous system. Psychological factors may play a part in some people.

Infections, e.g. balanitis, are common in people with poorly controlled diabetes and can cause malaise, local pain and anxiety, which may all contribute to worsening erectile dysfunction.

Some drugs taken by people with diabetes, such as beta-blockers and thiazide diuretics used to treat hypertension, antidepressants and anxiolytic agents are associated with erectile dysfunction. Alcohol in excess may also cause erectile dysfunction.

Taking a history and examination
This needs to be done in a relaxed environment (Table 24).

History
Questions that can be asked to elicit information are:
- Is there a lack of libido?
- Is there a problem with getting an erection?
- Do early morning erections still occur?
- Are there ejaculation problems?
- Any recent change of sexual partner?
- How important is the erectile dysfunction to them and their partner?
- What tablets are they taking?
- How much alcohol are they drinking?

Examination
Genitalia, cardiovascular system and peripheral nervous system.

Treatment of erectile dysfunction
General measures
Withdraw any drugs that may be contributing to the problem. Modify alcohol intake if necessary. Improve diabetes control. Counselling and advice to both partners.

Pharmacological therapy
- MUSE. This involves the intraurethral administration of prostaglandin E_1 using a specially designed introducer that the person themselves can administer.
- Intracavernosal injections of vasoactive drugs. Direct injection of vasoactive drugs into the corpus cavernosa of the penis can be an effective way of producing an erection. The most commonly used drug is prostaglandin E_1. The main

Table 24. Distinguishing between psychological and organic causes

	Psychological	Organic
Onset	often sudden	gradual
Permanence	intermittent or partial	total
Nocturnal erections	sometimes	never
Psychological symptoms	present	absent
Other microvascular complications	often absent	present
Erection lost on penetration	often happens	no erections

problem with this form of treatment, as with MUSE, is overcoming the difficulties and barriers that people may have to injecting into the penis or introducing something into the urethra. Satisfaction with treatment rates can approach 75% initially but discontinuation rates approach 50%.[64,65]

- Oral therapy. The emergence of sildenafil as an oral treatment for erectile dysfunction has been an important breakthrough. It works by suppressing the enzyme phosphodiesterase type 5 (PDE5), which occurs naturally in the erectile tissue of the penis. PDE5 breaks down intracellular guanosine monophosphate (cGMP), which is produced during arousal and causes the vascular changes that lead to erection of the penis.

  Sildenafil is taken an hour or so before intended intercourse. It does not by itself produce arousal, but allows an erection to occur during sexual foreplay. It is available in 25, 50 or 100 mg tablets. The stronger doses are needed in people with diabetes and a response rate of up to 60% has been reported.[66]

  Two other PDE5 inhibitors have now been released. One is tadalafil and the other vardenafil.

  PDE5 inhibitors can interact with nitrate-containing medications to cause hypotension so they should not be used

Erectile dysfunction diagnosis and management summary

Responsibilities of family physician

- ask about any problems at annual review
- ask about symptoms of erectile dysfunction
- physiological or psychological?
  – ask appropriate questions

if physiological

- offer an oral agent and titrate to maximum dose
- offer therapy
- if not effective offer other options
  – injection therapy or vacuum devices
- review and follow up

in people with ischaemic heart disease who are taking nitrate therapy.

- Vacuum tumescence devices. These consist of cylinders into which the penis is placed, and from which air is removed creating a vacuum, which produces an erection. They can be very effective and are free of systemic side effects. There are however difficulties in getting over the obvious problems of patient education, and some decide that this treatment is not acceptable for them.
- Surgical procedures. It may be necessary to operate to correct anatomical penile abnormalities resulting from phimosis and Peyronie's disease.

  It may also be possible to implant a penile prosthesis in people who do not respond to other treatment modalities.

Metabolic syndrome

It is now well recognized that there is a strong linkage between Type 2 diabetes and coronary artery disease. In addition, this linkage or risk probably precedes the actual diagnosis of Type 2 diabetes as people with the state of impaired glucose tolerance (IGT) have a greater risk of coronary disease than those with normal glucose tolerance. The metabolic syndrome is a constellation of abnormalities, each of which carry a risk for coronary artery disease and collectively increase that risk (Tables 25 and 26).[67] Insulin resistance is an essential component of the metabolic syndrome and it is associated with hyperinsulinaemia, dyslipidaemia, essential hypertension, abdominal obesity, and glucose intolerance or Type 2 diabetes.[68,69] Not uncommonly other abnormalities are identified in patients with metabolic syndrome. These include blood coagulation abnormalities – increased plasminogen activator inhibitor type 1 (PAI-1) and increased fibrinogen levels. Microalbuminuria and hyperuricaemia are also commonly associated.

Table 25. Features of the metabolic syndrome

- insulin resistance
- hyperinsulinaemia
- dyslipidaemia
  - low HDL; increased triglycerides; increased small-density particle LDL
- essential hypertension
- abdominal obesity
- glucose intolerance/Type 2 diabetes
- blood coagulation abnormalities
  - increased PAI-1; increased fibrogen levels
- hyperuricaemia
- microalbuminuria

Table 26. Identification of the metabolic syndrome*

At least three of the following abnormalities:

Waist circumference	>102 cm (men)
	>88 cm (women)
Serum triglycerides	>1.7 mmol/l
Serum HDL cholesterol	<1.05 mmol/l (men)
	<1.03 mmol/l (women)
Blood pressure	≥ 130/85 mmHg
Serum fasting glucose	6.1–7.0 mmol/l

* Executive Summary of The Third Report of The National Cholesterol Education Program (NCEP) Expert Panel on Detection, Evaluation, And Treatment of High Blood Cholesterol In Adults (Adult Treatment Panel III). *JAMA* 2001; **285**(19): 2486–97.

The obesity is characterized by an increase in visceral fat, which appears to be metabolically active. In addition, the visceral obesity is closely associated with increased cardiovascular risk.[70]

Dyslipidaemia is similarly characterized by lower high-density lipoprotein (HDL) cholesterol levels, an increase in atherogenic low-density lipoprotein (LDL), and elevated triglyceride levels. In the presence of insulin resistance, there is increased output of free fatty acids which, in turn, may play a role in the associated abnormalities of decreased pancreatic insulin secretion, increased hepatic glucose production and decreased glucose uptake.

Hypertension is another key component of the metabolic syndrome and is closely associated with insulin resistance and hyperinsulinaemia.[71] Essential hypertension is one of the earliest signals of the metabolic syndrome.

Impaired glucose tolerance or Type 2 diabetes is another important component of the metabolic syndrome. Once again there is a clear association between these abnormalities and coronary artery disease and both are associated with the state of visceral obesity and insulin resistance.

Increased levels of PAI-1 are associated both with the metabolic syndrome and increased risk of coronary artery disease. There is a common linkage between PAI-1 abnormalities, visceral obesity and insulin resistance. Similarly, hyperuricaemia is commonly seen in patients with metabolic syndrome and is linked with the clinical manifestations of metabolic syndrome – hypertension, glucose intolerance and dyslipidaemia.

Patients with metabolic syndrome may be at a similar risk of developing coronary disease, as those with Type 2 diabetes.[72]

Treatment

The goal of treatment in metabolic syndrome is to reduce cardiovascular risk. This involves treating the aetiological factors of the metabolic syndrome and the individual risk factors of hypertension, glucose intolerance or diabetes, and dyslipidaemia.

A reduction in obesity has beneficial effects on all risk factors. Thus, the concept of an appropriate diet linked with a weight-reducing exercise programme can prove to be most beneficial. Drug therapy utilizing weight-reducing drugs such as orlistat and sibutramine may provide weight loss benefit, improve the metabolic status of the diabetic patient, and help prevent diabetes in obese subjects.[73–75]

Reducing insulin resistance may prove to be extremely beneficial in treating the metabolic syndrome. New drugs such as the thiazolidinediones (TZDs) have been shown to reduce insulin resistance in patients with impaired carbohydrate tolerance and in those with Type 2 diabetes. Clinical studies with rosiglitazone and pioglitazone have further shown improvement in many of the individual risk factors associated with the metabolic syndrome. It is possible, that these drugs may prove to have a powerful role in the prevention and treatment of coronary artery disease by treating all the components of the metabolic syndrome, as well as insulin resistance.

Aggressive management of carbohydrate intolerance or diabetes, will lead to improvement in carbohydrate metabolism and thus reduce cardiovascular risk. As glucose levels fall, triglyceride values will decrease, which may also decrease cardiovascular risk.

Aggressive management of hypertension has also proven to be beneficial with reduction of blood pressure to levels of 130/80 mmHg or less providing a major benefit.[49,76]

The results of prospective lipid-lowering trials have proven the benefit of statin therapy. Studies such as 4S,[77] the Heart Protection Study[78] and ASCOT[79] have demonstrated both direct and indirect benefits in terms of lowering lipid values and reducing cardiovascular risk.[77,78]

There is increasing recognition that the dyslipidaemia associated with diabetes is a key factor in the development of coronary artery disease. Results from several major clinical studies have suggested that the presence of diabetes constitutes a major risk factor for coronary artery disease and thus the dyslipidaemia must be treated aggressively.

The Heart Protection Study emphasized the benefit of lowering the LDL cholesterol levels in the diabetic patient and adds confirmation to previous reports that diabetes constitutes a major risk for cardiovascular disease. The Framingham Study risk equations are valuable in calculating cardiovascular risk assessment in the non-diabetic patient, but the actual calculation can be time-consuming and thus difficult to implement within the context of a busy physician's clinic.

With the increasing consensus that the diabetic patient must have abnormal lipid values treated more aggressively, clinical guidelines are recommending that LDL-cholesterol should be lowered to at least below levels of 2.5 mmol/l (Table 27).[67]

Table 27. Target goals of management of lipid abnormalities		
LDL cholesterol		**Total/HDL cholesterol**
mmol/l	**and**	ratio
<2.5		<4.0

Table 28. Recommended targets for glucose control

	HbA$_{1c}$	Fasting/ preprandial glucose	2-hour postprandial glucose
Target	<7%	4–7 mmol/l	5–10 mmol/l

It is clear that an aggressive management programme must be undertaken in a patient with metabolic syndrome and especially in those who have exhibited carbohydrate intolerance or Type 2 diabetes. In many respects, the treatment of diabetes is no longer the treatment of glucose alone, but a treatment of three key risk factors: abnormal glucose levels, hypertension, and dyslipidaemia.

Managing the carbohydrate intolerance

This topic has been discussed in previous sections (pages 29–58) and the drugs used to achieve specific targets have been fully reviewed. As more clinical research data become available, glucose targets may become lower so that the HbA$_{1c}$ is < 7% and in fact could ideally be closer to 6–6.5%. Postprandial glucoses, which may also be linked to cardiovascular disease, should be kept within the range of 5–10 mmol/l (Table 28).

Management of hypertension

The goal in managing blood pressure is to bring the values to less than 140/80 mmHg (Table 29). Indeed many international therapeutic guidelines recommend a blood pressure goal of less than 130/80 mmHg in the diabetic patient. There is now

Table 29. Goals of management of hypertension

Hypertensive patient with diabetes
less than 140/80 mmHg
Hypertensive patient with diabetes and proteinuria > 1.0 g/day
less than 135/75 mmHg

excellent evidence that the ACE inhibitors or angiotensin II receptor antagonists (AIIRAs) are of benefit to the diabetic patient. Important prospective clinical trials have shown the renal protective effect of the AIIRAs and ACE inhibitors.[76,80–84] These should be considered as first-line therapy, but it is likely that most hypertensive diabetic patients will require at least two or three medications to lower their blood pressure to target. The use of a diuretic should be considered early in the treatment programme utilizing either low-dose bendrofluazide or indapamide. In those patients who are resistant to treatment, furosemide in relatively high doses may be required. Other agents such as a dihydropyridine calcium-channel blocker, the alpha-blocker doxasosin and/or a beta-blocker can be added to achieve target values.

The publication of the Steno II paper[85] has further emphasized the need to aggressively treat all cardiovascular risk factors. This target-driven, long-term study intensively treating all multiple risk factors in Type 2 diabetic patients, resulted in a 50% decrease in the risk of cardiovascular and microvascular events.

The use of aspirin therapy in diabetes

The diabetic patient is at increased risk of cardiovascular disease and vascular thrombosis. A major contributor to the increased risk is an abnormality in platelet function. It has been found that platelets in diabetic patients demonstrate increased sensitivity to platelet aggravating agents. Aspirin has been found to block this mechanism and has been suggested as both primary and secondary prevention for cardiovascular events in the diabetic patient. Aspirin therapy should be considered in all diabetic patients who have evidence of large vessel disease, those who have coronary artery disease, peripheral vascular disease, and previous episodes of stroke or transient ischaemic attack.

Aspirin should also be considered in those who are at high risk of development of vascular complications.[86] This would include those with a family history of coronary artery disease, hypertension, dyslipidaemia, obesity and those who smoke.

Table 30. Recommendations for aspirin use

1. *As a primary prevention strategy in diabetics with high-risk characteristics*
- family history of coronary artery disease
- hypertension
- obesity
- dyslipidaemia
- cigarette smoking
2. *As a secondary prevention strategy in those who have previous evidence of large vessel disease*

Thus, aspirin therapy is recommended for most Type 2 diabetic patients and those with metabolic syndrome (Table 30). UK guidelines recommend adding aspirin in primary prevention if CHD risk is 15% or greater.

Dosage

Use enteric-coated aspirin. The recommended preventive doses vary in different countries. In the UK a dose of 75 mg daily is usually used and sometimes increased to 150 mg daily, however, in some countries the dose used may be as high as 325 mg.

Aspirin should not be used in those at risk of bleeding or with aspirin allergy. Nor should aspirin be used in patients under the age of 21 because of the increased risk of Reye's syndrome.

In the UK, guidelines suggest not to use aspirin in uncontrolled hypertension.

Hypoglycaemia

Hypoglycaemia is a state of abnormally low blood glucose. It is the single most important impediment to achieving ideal glucose control, particularly in the Type 1 diabetic patient.[87] Because severe hypoglycaemia can lead to a serious decrease in cognitive function, glucose levels are often maintained at higher values to prevent the occurrence of hypoglycaemia. This defeats the very purpose of trying to treat diabetes when better glucose control can lead to a decrease in the vascular complications associated with diabetes. New clinical guidelines for the management of diabetes are recommending even lower targets with HbA_{1c} values between 6 and 6.5%. As HbA_{1c} targets are lowered, there is an increased risk of hypoglycaemia.

Definition of hypoglycaemia

There is no precise definition of hypoglycaemia, as patients may experience symptoms of hypoglycaemia at differing levels of glucose (Table 31). Clinical hypoglycaemia can be defined by a series of specific events:

1. Development of autonomic or neuroglycopenic symptoms.
2. Measurement of a low plasma glucose.
3. Relief of symptoms following the ingestion of carbohydrate.

While a precise glucose level cannot be used as a definition, certain physiologic changes take place as glucose levels fall. As plasma glucose falls below 4.0 mmol/l there is a release of a series of counter-regulatory hormones including cortisol, glucagon, adrenaline (epinephrine) and growth hormone. As the glucose falls lower to levels below 3.0 mmol/l neurogenic (autonomic) and later neuroglycopenic symptoms will occur. A loss of cognitive function will also occur, as glucose levels fall below 2.5 mmol/l. There is considerable variation among diabetic patients, as to when, if at all, these symptoms will occur in relationship to specific plasma glucose levels.

Another useful way to define hypoglycaemia describes the ability of the patient to respond to the low sugars.

Table 31. Symptoms of hypoglycaemia

Autonomic (neurogenic)
- tingling of extremities particularly fingertips, nose tip, and lips
- anxiety
- sweating
- trembling
- palpitations
- hunger and/or nausea

Neuroglycopenic
- decreased ability to concentrate
- weakness
- vision changes including double or blurred vision
- confusion
- difficulty in formulating words
- fatigue
- dizziness and/or headache
- drowsiness

In the presence of mild hypoglycaemia, the patient may experience the autonomic symptoms associated with hypoglycaemia and is then able to treat the event to prevent a further fall of plasma glucose. During moderate hypoglycaemia the patient may experience both autonomic and neuroglycopenic-mediated symptoms, but is still able to self-treat the hypoglycaemic event.

With severe hypoglycaemia, the patient will require the assistance of another person to treat the event. The event is marked by serious mental confusion and the patient may lapse into an unconscious state. During that time, the patient may come to physical harm, may vomit and aspirate, or experience a seizure.

Hypoglycaemia unawareness is a serious situation that places the patient at considerable risk. Inevitably, it leads to a failure to achieve satisfactory glucose control. The patient will experience neuroglycopenic symptoms including confusion and loss of consciousness before experiencing the warning symptoms normally provided by the autonomic response to hypoglycaemia. In effect, the patient may have no warning of the impending hypoglycaemic event. The presence of hypoglycaemia unawareness can lead to major restrictions in lifestyle and place the patient in constant danger.[88]

Other factors contribute to the development of hypoglycaemia unawareness. The response of glucagon to hypoglycaemia is decreased within a few years of the diagnosis of Type 1 diabetes and thus decreases a major protective mechanism against hypoglycaemia. There may also be a general loss of other counter-regulatory hormones contributing to the lack of a corrective response to hypoglycaemia.[89]

There is a benefit in reducing or eliminating events of hypoglycaemia, as defective glucose hormone counter regulation appears to be reversible. As hypoglycaemic events are reduced, there is an overall improvement in the ability of the patient to recognize a hypoglycaemic event.[90,91]

Long-term complications of severe and repeated hypoglycaemia

The major complication related to repeated and severe hypoglycaemia relates to changes in intellectual capacity. There is a concern that repeated events of hypoglycaemia may lead to intellectual impairment and general loss of cognitive function. Fortunately, this appears to be rare in the adult,[92,93] but there may be greater risk for the child with diabetes who is also at a greater risk of repeated and severe hypoglycaemia.[94] Persistent neurological deficits such as hemiparesis are rare and may be more related to injury sustained during the hypoglycaemic event or an associated seizure. Also, there is an association between repeated hypoglycaemia and the development of hypoglycaemia unawareness.[93]

Perhaps one of the more serious sequelae of repeated and severe hypoglycaemia are the changes that will be imposed upon the patient who is experiencing repeated hypoglycaemic events. The patient's daily routine will be disrupted and some work and leisure activities denied. The patient's driving licence

Table 32. Risk factors for severe hypoglycaemia

- low HbA_{1c} (generally less than 6%)
- insulin use
- hypoglycaemia unawareness
- duration of diabetes
- previous or multiple episodes of severe hypoglycaemia
- autonomic neuropathy
- adolescents are at increased risk

may have to be suspended or withdrawn. The patient must be counselled to self-glucose monitor throughout the day and particularly at times of increased danger. These would include driving a car, work-related dangers, swimming and other water activities, or being in a situation where the patient is responsible for the safety of others.

Insulin therapy and hypoglycaemia

The major Diabetes Control and Complications Trial (DCCT)[36] demonstrated the benefit of intensive insulin therapy using either a multi-dose insulin therapy programme or pump therapy. A significant decrease in microvascular complications among Type 1 diabetics receiving intensive therapy compared with a controlled conservative-managed group, was a major finding from the study. Similar benefits are probably present for the Type 2 diabetic patient on insulin who uses an intensive-insulin therapy programme.

The intensively treated group in the DCCT, however, had a three-fold increase in the events of hypoglycaemia compared with the conventionally treated group. As their HbA_{1c} was lowered within the study, the risk of hypoglycaemia increased.

This risk of hypoglycaemia is also present in the Type 2 patient treated with insulin. Clinical studies have suggested that if intensive insulin management is accompanied by a complete and thorough educational programme, the risk of hypoglycaemia decreases.[95]

The use of new insulins may also decrease the risk of hypoglycaemia in both Type 1 and Type 2 diabetes (see Section: Insulin, pages 36–58).

Role of animal or human insulins in precipitating hypoglycaemia

Shortly after the introduction of human insulins, there was a concern that there may be an increased risk of hypoglycaemia with human insulin compared with animal-prepared insulin. Numerous studies have reviewed this issue and there is no clear evidence that there is an increased risk when using human insulin.[96,97]

Hypoglycaemia induced by oral antihyperglycaemic agents

Hypoglycaemia induced by oral antihyperglycaemic agents is in fact more common than with the use of insulin.[37] Severe hypoglycaemia is rare, but many patients may not recognize the symptoms of hypoglycaemia and this can contribute to the general state of ill health in many Type 2 diabetic patients. Elderly patients are particularly vulnerable as they are at increased risk of hypoglycaemia, and hypoglycaemia symptoms may be attributed to other illnesses or even ignored. The actual incidence of hypoglycaemia is probably underestimated, as the events are often undetected or not reported.

Of the oral drugs, the insulin-stimulating drugs are the most likely to cause hypoglycaemia. These include the sulphonylureas, meglitinides (repaglinide), and amino acid derivatives (nateglinide). The longer-acting sulphonylureas are more likely to induce hypoglycaemia and this group includes glibenclamide (glyburide) and chlorpropamide.[98] The shorter-acting sulphonylureas, such as gliclazide, glimepiride, as well as repaglinide, and nateglinide are less likely to cause hypoglycaemia. This particular benefit is most apparent during the first year of treatment.[98–100]

The frequency of hypoglycaemia is less in three classes of oral antihyperglycaemic drugs:

- Alpha-glucosidase inhibitors (acarbose).[42,46]

Table 33. Drugs contributing to hypoglycaemia

- high-dose salicylates
- beta-blockers
- sulphonamide antibiotics
- warfarin
- phenylbutazone
- tricyclic antidepressants
- paracetamol (acetaminophen)
- fibrates
- ACE inhibitors

- Biguanides (metformin).[101]
- Thiazolidinediones (rosiglitazone, pioglitazone).[42]

If these drugs are combined with an insulin-stimulating drug or insulin, there is of course an increased risk of hypoglycaemia. For the patient on an alpha-glucosidase inhibitor, it is important to use glucose when treating hypoglycaemia rather than a sucrose or starch, because of the delayed absorption of these sugars.

Some drugs, commonly used in the treatment of other medical disorders, can contribute to hypoglycaemic events (Table 33).

Medical factors precipitating hypoglycaemia

Several other factors may be predominant in causing hypoglycaemia (Table 34). Older patients are more prone to hypoglycaemia often because of inappropriate drug use and dosage, and also because they may frequently miss a meal when taking a drug, such as an insulin-stimulating agent. Patients with impaired renal or liver function may have prolonged action of insulin or an oral antihyperglycaemic agent. Patients with loss of cortisol secretion, such as in adrenal insufficiency, or with significant gastrointestinal disease are also more prone to hypoglycaemia. Alcohol will prevent production of new glucose formation to overcome a current or an impending

Table 34. Factors that increase risk of hypoglycaemia

- the older patient
- impaired renal or liver function
- gastrointestinal disease
- adrenal insufficiency
- missed or delayed meals
- alcohol consumption
- exercise
- drug therapies
  - oral antihyperglycaemic agents
  - insulin
- dementia and certain neurological disorders, e.g. stroke

hypoglycaemic event and thus can precipitate hypoglycaemia or prevent recovery from hypoglycaemia. Exercise and missed or delayed meals will contribute to hypoglycaemia in all age groups.

Exercise and hypoglycaemia

For the patient on insulin or an insulin-stimulating agent, there is a risk of hypoglycaemia associated with exercise. The timing of the hypoglycaemic event associated with exercise can differ between individuals and with different exercise routines. Hypoglycaemia may be experienced during the exercise programme or within a short time of its completion, but can also occur many hours after exercise has been completed. The use of fast-acting insulin analogues reduces the risk of hypoglycaemia after exercise, as does the use of "low-risk" antihyperglycaemic agents in the Type 2 diabetic patient.

Decreasing the risk of hypoglycaemia

Oral antihyperglycaemic agents

For the person at greater risk of hypoglycaemia, insulin-stimulating drugs should be avoided and either an alpha-glucosidase inhibitor, and/or a thiazolidinedione, and/or metformin used. If an insulin-stimulating drug is required, then shorter-acting drugs such as repaglinide, nateglinide, gliclazide, or glimepiride, should be used.

Insulin

All patients on an intensive insulin regimen should have received a comprehensive education programme reviewing aspects of glucose monitoring, insulin adjustment and the impact of exercise, diet, and changes in daily events. If a hypoglycaemic event has occurred, the cause and management of each event should be reviewed by the diabetes education team. A fast-acting insulin analogue is preferred to soluble (regular) insulin as the pre-meal bolus insulin. The pre-supper use of an insulin analogue, rather than using soluble insulin, may also reduce the risk of nocturnal hypoglycaemia.

Administering a basal isophane (NPH) insulin dose at bedtime rather than suppertime may also further reduce the risk of nocturnal hypoglycaemia. Insulin glargine provides an even greater reduction of nocturnal hypoglycaemic risk compared with isophane insulin.

Patients with multiple risk factors for severe hypoglycaemia should be counselled on how to develop strategies to decrease the risk of severe hypoglycaemia. This is particularly important in those patients with hypoglycaemia unawareness. Specific strategies that might benefit these patients include:

1. More frequent use of glucose monitoring with appropriate adjustments of insulin at times of identified hypoglycaemia.
2. Increasing the number of insulin injections with lower insulin doses.
3. Raising glucose targets.

For the exercising patient who is at increased risk of hypoglycaemia, it is important to review all aspects of the exercise programme, diet, and impact of food and insulin. At the beginning of a new exercise routine, self-glucose monitoring should be performed before and if possible during a prolonged exercise period. Glucose measurements should also be taken after exercise and for many hours after completion of the exercise programme. If pre-exercise glucose levels are below

5 mmol/l, patients on insulin or insulin-stimulating agents will require some rapidly absorbed carbohydrates before commencing their exercise programme.

If the patient is on insulin then they should be advised to inject the insulin distant from the exercising limbs.

Treatment of hypoglycaemia

In the presence of hypoglycaemia, the goal is to elevate the blood glucose to a safer level and decrease the risk to the diabetic patient. At the same time, the amount of glucose provided to treat the event, should not lead to excessively high plasma glucose levels. Because of the varying absorption properties of different carbohydrates, it is preferable to use a simple glucose as the means of raising the blood glucose during hypoglycaemia. The use of a monosaccharide glucose substance (15 g) will produce a rise in blood glucose of approximately 1.0 mmol/l within 20 minutes of ingestion, thus providing relief for most patients. An increased dose of 20 g of oral glucose will elevate blood glucose by approximately 3.6 mmol/l. Orange juice and glucose gels provide a much slower glucose rise. In the semiconscious or unconscious patient, the use of buccal glucose gels does not provide an adequate increase in serum glucose due to the poor absorption of glucose through the buccal mucosa.[88,102]

In the unconscious patient, there is some urgency in ensuring that blood glucose levels are raised. If there is not easy access to more sophisticated medical help, the injection of 1.0 mg of glucagon will produce a glucose rise from 3–12 mmol/l within 1 hour.[103] Ideally, the "at-risk" patient's partner or care giver, should be trained in advance as to how to administer the glucagon injection. If available, trained personnel should give an intravenous infusion of glucose. Once the patient is conscious, further carbohydrate can be provided orally.

Severe hypoglycaemia induced by sulphonylurea ingestion may be prolonged and a constant infusion of glucose may be required to provide a recovery.[104]

Treating hypoglycaemia

For mild to moderate hypoglycaemia

- 15 g of glucose in the form of glucose tablets
- repeat after 15 minutes if the blood glucose remains less than 4.0 mmol/l

In the conscious patient with severe hypoglycaemia

- 20 g of carbohydrate in the form of glucose tablets
- Repeat after 15 minutes if blood glucose remains less than 4.0 mmol/l

In the unconscious patient with severe hypoglycaemia

- Patient is not close to a hospital – 1.0 mg of subcutaneous or intramuscular glucagon
- In the hospital setting use intravenous glucose 10–25 g given over 3 minutes

For the patient taking an alpha glucosidase inhibitor experiencing hypoglycaemia

- Use glucose tablets rather than sucrose or a starch to reverse hypoglycaemia

Ensure that all episodes of severe hypoglycaemia are reviewed and discussed with the patient to help identify the cause of the event and prevent future episodes.

Hyperglycaemic diabetic emergencies

There are two hyperglycaemic diabetic emergencies that, while not common, are associated with high mortality: diabetic ketoacidosis (DKA) and non-ketotic hyperosmolar state, more commonly referred to as the hyperosmolar, hyperglycaemic state (HHS) or hyperosmolar, non-ketotic coma (HONK). Mortality rates for DKA can reach 10% and for HHS can be as high as 50%.[105] In an older group of patients, mortality rates for these two conditions may in fact be similar. While there has always been a distinction between DKA and HHS, it is likely that both disorders can present with degrees of concurrent ketoacidosis and hyperosmolarity.[106]

Pathophysiology

The metabolic abnormalities associated with DKA and HHS result from an absolute or relative insulin deficiency and the release of counter-regulatory hormones. As the disorder develops, counter-regulatory hormones will lead to increased hepatic glucose output and decreased glucose uptake, resulting in hyperglycaemia. As glucose levels rise, there will be increased urinary loss of glucose, subsequent dehydration and eventually decreased kidney perfusion and glucose output, with increasing hyperglycaemia.

The low insulin levels and elevated levels of counter-regulatory hormones also lead to fat cell breakdown and the release of free fatty acids. These free fatty acids will eventually be converted to ketone bodies in the form of beta-hydroxybutyric acid and acetoacetic acid. The ketotic state is most commonly associated with DKA and only rarely seen in HHS. The increasing acidosis leads to a fall in serum bicarbonate levels and this can be measured by calculating the anion gap (Table 35).

In the presence of acidosis, the anion gap will increase. Generally, beta-hydroxybutyric acid levels are higher than acetoacetic acid levels and during the development of DKA,

Table 35. Calculating the anion gap

Use the following formula with standard electrolyte measurements

$[Na^+] - ([Cl^-] + [HCO^-])$ Normal Anion Gap = 12 mmol/l

DKA > 12 mmol/l

this difference will be increased. Some methodologies measuring the presence of ketones may not detect beta-hydroxybutyric acid and only measure the acetoacetic acid levels, thus underestimating the degree of ketosis. A bedside meter analysis that measures blood beta-hydroxybutyric acid is now available and can provide a rapid reporting of the degree of ketosis allowing assessment of treatment progress.[107]

Fluid and electrolyte losses

During the osmotic diuresis induced by the high glucose levels, there will be severe fluid and electrolyte losses. Fluid losses in DKA range between 5 and 7 litres and in HHS, 7 and 12 litres. Associated with the fluid loss will be a major loss of both sodium and potassium. Because of the osmotic shifts of water occurring with both DKA and HHS, the plasma sodium concentration needs to be corrected for the concurrent hyperglycaemia (Table 36).

In both DKA and HHS there can be extensive loss of total body potassium. Because of the shift of water and potassium between the intracellular and extracellular space, the laboratory measurement of serum potassium may be normal or even elevated at the time of the first assessment. As long as the osmotic diuresis continues, there will be excessive urinary potassium loss, requiring aggressive replacement.

Table 36. Estimating plasma sodium concentration levels

For every 5.6 mmol/l increase in glucose above 5.6 mmol/l, add 1.6 mmol to the laboratory reported sodium level

Table 37. Causes of DKA and HHS

DKA	HHS
infection	infection
omission of insulin injection	undiagnosed Type 2 diabetes
inadequate insulin injection	cerebrovascular accident
previously undiagnosed Type 1 diabetes	myocardial infarction
	acute pancreatitis
	drug-induced hyperglycaemia:
	– steroids
	– thiazide diuretics
	– phenytoin

Presentation and assessment of DKA and HHS

The key to the management of DKA and HHS is a rapid clinical assessment accompanied by instant action (Table 37).[108]

DKA generally occurs in the younger patient with Type 1 diabetes and the history of the event will be short. Clinical features of dehydration are usually present. Abdominal pain associated with nausea and vomiting may lead to the mistaken diagnosis of an acute abdominal emergency. There may be physical signs of a generalized or localized infection. The patient may also present with deep and rapid respirations with a strong odour of acetone, so-called Kussmaul-Kien respiration.

The patient presenting with HHS is generally older, obese, and the history may extend for days or weeks prior to the presentation. The degree of dehydration in HHS may be far more severe than DKA and the patient may be exhibiting signs of vascular collapse. Abdominal pain may also be present, as well as signs of generalized or local infection.

Laboratory results in DKA and HHS[109]

Generally the degree of hyperglycaemia is far greater in HHS compared with DKA. In fact, the degree of hyperglycaemia in

Table 38. Calculation of serum osmolality

$(2\times$ serum $Na^+) +$ serum glucose

Normal $= 219$ mmol/kg H_2O

Definition of HHS: > 320 mmol/kg H_2O

DKA may not be excessively high while the degree of ketosis is profound. HHS can be diagnosed on the basis of the serum osmolality (Table 38). DKA can be further differentiated by pH ≤ 7.3 and this is commonly associated with a decrease in bicarbonate to < 15 mmol/l.

The blood leukocyte count may often be increased as a result of infection and also from the stress and dehydration associated with the condition. An ECG should be done immediately upon admission, with careful assessment of the T-wave formation, which may indicate the presence of hyperkalaemia or hypokalaemia. The ECG provides an "early warning system" for hypokalaemia allowing for immediate replacement of potassium, even before the laboratory potassium value becomes available (Tables 39 and 40).

Table 39. Essential laboratory assessment in DKA and HHS

- serum glucose
- serum electrolytes
- serum osmolality
- blood pH
- white blood cell count
- ECG
- blood/urine culture
- chest X-ray

Table 40. Comparison of diagnostic laboratory criteria for DKA and HHS

Laboratory measurement	Normal values	DKA	HHS
glucose mmol/l	<7.0	>14.0	>34.0
arterial pH	7.35–7.45	<7.3	>7.3
serum bicarbonate (mmol/l)	22–28	<15.0	>15.0
serum osmolality (mmol/kg H_2O)	275–295	<320.0	>320.0
anion gap (mmol/l)	<12.0	>12.0	high or low

Clinical management

The key to successful management and reduced morbidity and mortality depends on the correction of dehydration, hyperglycaemia, electrolyte deficiencies, and acidosis. The rapid identification of the precipitating illness is essential.[109] Clinical assessments should be made every 30 minutes and then hourly until the extreme conditions have been corrected. Monitoring should then take place every 2 to 4 hours until the condition has resolved. Electrolytes should be monitored every 1 to 2 hours and glucose meter readings taken on an hourly basis.

Fluid replacement
- First hour: 1.0–1.5 litres of isotonic saline (0.9% sodium chloride)
- Second hour: Reassess state of hydration (blood pressure, urine output), and
  – If severe dehydration continues: 1.0 litre of isotonic saline
  – If hydration improves: 500–750 ml (0.45% sodium chloride)
- When plasma glucose less than 12 mmol/l: iv fluid should contain 5% dextrose
- Watch for over-hydration

Potassium replacement
- Ensure adequate urine output before replacing potassium
- Infuse 20–30 mmol of potassium to each litre of infusion fluid to maintain potassium concentrations between 4–5 mmol/l
- In the presence of inverted T-waves or a serum potassium less than 3.3 mmol/l commence immediate potassium replacement
- Delay insulin therapy until potassium concentration greater than 3.3 mmol/l to avoid cardiac abnormalities
- Monitor serum potassium every 1 to 2 hours during the first 5 hours; measure every 4 to 6 hours as required thereafter

Insulin therapy
- Utilize low-dose insulin infusion
- Commence iv insulin infusion rate at 0.1 unit/kg/hour
- Monitor serum glucose hourly
- Double insulin infusion if glucose fall is < 3 mmol/l/hour
- Continue insulin infusion until resolution of DKA or HHS
- Commence subcutaneous insulin therapy as iv insulin therapy is decreased and stopped

While deficiencies of bicarbonate and phosphates have been identified, replacement has not been found to be beneficial and is not recommended.

Long-term follow up

This is an essential component of treatment. The aetiology of the DKA or HHS must be carefully identified and then discussed with the patient. To avoid a recurrence, the precipitating events and clinical presentation of the illness must also be reviewed with the patient. A specific educational program can then be set in place to help the patient understand how the event could be prevented on a future occasion. If a precipitating event has been identified it should be adequately treated and measures taken, if possible, to prevent its re-occurrence.

Diabetes in pregnancy

Perhaps one of the most important topics related to diabetes treatment is the management of the pregnancy in the woman with diabetes. There is a need for comprehensive care preconception, during the pregnancy, and into the postpartum period. The diabetic pregnancy is associated with an increased risk of many complications (Table 41). The dominant issue becomes one of maintaining perfect glucose control before and after conception. By achieving ideal glucose management, the risks to the foetus and the mother are greatly reduced. The incidence of these complications of the diabetes pregnancy can be decreased when glucose targets are achieved.[110–117]

Management prior to conception

The preconception diabetes management programme actually begins as the diabetic woman enters childbearing age. Even a brief chat during regular clinic visits about the importance of good glucose control during a pregnancy sets the stage for the later intensive treatment of the diabetic pregnancy. An ideal time to discuss pregnancy will be when the diabetic woman seeks advice about contraception. Discussions concerning the eventual timing and planning of her pregnancy, as well as contraception, help emphasize the important issue of ideal glucose control, both prior to conception and during the pregnancy (Table 42).

Table 41. Complications of the diabetic pregnancy

- congenital abnormalities
- spontaneous abortion
- accelerated hypertension
- pre-eclampsia
- progression of vascular complications – nephropathy/retinopathy
- birth trauma

Table 42. Preconception issues

Early discussion
- planning
- establish glucose goals
- contraception
- multiple team involvement
- dietary advice

Full medical assessment
- history
- examination
- blood pressure
- retinal review
- laboratory assessments to include HbA_{1c}, protein excretion and TSH

Despite the clear advantage of good glucose control prior to conception, especially during the first 8 weeks of the pregnancy, the tragedy is that many diabetic women are first assessed after conception. Many of these women have Type 2 diabetes, are treated with oral agents, and most frequently are not in ideal control. With the steady increase in the incidence of Type 2 diabetes among young people this trend will likely increase.[118,119] A concerted effort is thus required on the part of all primary care givers, physicians and educators, to alert and inform the diabetic woman that there is tremendous advantage in planning a pregnancy and achieving target glucose values.

For the Type 1 woman with diabetes, planning should commence at least 3 months prior to the intended pregnancy. As oral contraceptives may alter insulin requirements, these drugs should be stopped 3 months prior to the pregnancy and the woman provided with barrier methods of contraception. At the same time, insulin doses will need to be adjusted to achieve the glucose target values that will be required during the pregnancy.

Women with Type 2 diabetes are most likely to be on oral agents. These drugs should be stopped at least 3 months prior to the intended pregnancy and glucose levels evaluated quickly. It is most likely that insulin will be required prior to the pregnancy and thus she will enter the pregnant stage with well-controlled glucose levels and a stable insulin dose. If the diabetic woman has already entered pregnancy while on oral agents, these drugs should be stopped immediately and insulin therapy commenced. It is essential to rapidly achieve perfect control of the glucose levels as it is in the early weeks of pregnancy, that the risks of foetal malformation are the highest.

A multidisciplinary diabetes healthcare team is essential to achieve the goal of a well-managed pregnancy.[113,114] The team should be composed of an endocrinologist/internist; nurse and dietary educators; and an obstetrician. It is important to establish a good working relationship with members of the team prior to commencing the pregnancy and to ensure that all members of the team have agreed on the precise goals of the pregnancy.

Prior to conception a full medical assessment should be performed. A detailed history should be obtained to determine the current health status and drug treatment of the patient. A review of previous medical concerns and complications should be detailed, as well as the history of any previous pregnancy.

The physical examination should include an assessment of potential vascular complications as well as a review of self-glucose monitoring records.

A laboratory assessment should include measurement of HbA_{1c}, urine protein excretion, thyroid-stimulating hormone (TSH), and a glucose monitor/serum glucose comparison. Because progression of retinopathy during pregnancy has been observed, particularly in those with poor glycaemic control, retinal assessment by an ophthalmologist should be made prior to conception, during the first and third trimester and following delivery of the baby. Untreated hypertension may also lead to progression of retinopathy. Because both nephropathy and retinopathy can progress with uncontrolled hypertension, management of hypertension becomes an important component of the overall management programme.[120]

Children of diabetic women appear to have an increased risk of neural tube defects and thus the normal folic acid supplement should be increased to 1–5 mg per day prior to conception until approximately 12 weeks of gestation.[115,121]

ACE inhibitors have been associated with foetal development abnormalities and thus should be stopped prior to conception.[122] At the same time, blood pressure should be monitored carefully in case additional medications are required to maintain ideal blood pressure control.

The glucose target prior to conception for the woman with Type 1 or Type 2 diabetes is an HbA_{1c} less than 7%. At this level, there appears to be a decreased risk of the diabetes complications associated with pregnancy. Pre- and post-glucose targets, as listed in Table 43 should be achieved.[123]

The Type 2 patient on oral agents should be transferred onto an insulin regimen prior to conception and established glucose targets achieved.

Managing the pregnant diabetic patient

Nutrition

A reduced caloric intake is not recommended during the pregnancy. In many situations, an increased caloric intake is required for the nutritional needs of the mother and the foetus. It is important to avoid ketosis in the mother and this may require increased caloric intake throughout the day including the need for regular snacks between meals. If morning sickness is a problem, the mother should review these issues with the dietitian as caloric substitutes can be made to ensure sufficient food intake.[124–126]

Glycaemic control

Self-glucose monitoring becomes the key to achieving glycaemic targets outlined in Table 43. In the preconception

Table 43. Glucose targets during pre-conception and during pregnancy (mmol/l)	
Preprandial	< 5.3
1 hour postprandial	< 7.8
2 hour postprandial	< 6.7
HbA_{1c}	< 7% (ideally as close as possible to 6%)

phase and throughout the pregnancy, regular monitoring is recommended.[127] Generally, four or more blood glucose measurements a day are required, to include preprandial and 2-hour postprandial time periods. It is important to remember that during the first trimester, particularly in a Type 1 diabetic, the risk of hypoglycaemia is higher, thus these target values may not be attainable.[128]

During the first trimester, frequent glucose monitoring will help prevent hypoglycaemic events and during the second trimester, when insulin resistance is increasing, glucose monitoring will help establish the necessary corrections of the insulin dose.

Insulin resistance and insulin therapy

There are definitive changes in insulin resistance during the pregnancy management programme. In the preconception preparation time, oral contraceptives will have been stopped approximately 3 months prior to conception to allow stabilization of therapy. Thus, there may be a change in insulin dose due to the removal of the hormone therapy. In the first trimester there is often a blunting of the counter-regulatory hormones leading to an increased risk of hypoglycaemia. At approximately 18–20 weeks' gestation, however, a dramatic change will begin. Hormone production from the placenta will oppose the action of the injected insulin and at the same time placental-enzyme action will lead to increased destruction of the exogenous insulin. Thus, there will be an effective increase in insulin resistance and need for an increased insulin dose, which will continue until approximately 32–34 weeks' gestation, when insulin requirements will reach a plateau.

Thus, during the first trimester insulin requirements may actually fall slightly in some patients and then steadily increase throughout the second trimester. During the latter part of the third trimester, insulin requirements are generally stable and in fact, a decrease in insulin requirements may provide an "early warning" system that placental function is decreasing and there may be concerns for the foetus. Towards the end of the pregnancy many women cannot maintain a high caloric intake

---

Table 44. Changing insulin requirements during pregnancy

Pre-conception
- after stopping hormonal contraception

First trimester
- decreased counter-regulatory hormone action with increased risk of hypoglycaemia

Second trimester
- increasing insulin resistance with increasing insulin requirements

Third trimester
- stabilization of insulin requirements
- 5-10% decrease of insulin requirements requires increased foetal supervision

---

and insulin requirements may fall accordingly. A 5–10% decrease in insulin requirements in the latter part of the third trimester, would suggest the need for more intensive monitoring of the foetus (Table 44).

Multiple daily insulin injections are required for all Type 1 and many Type 2 diabetic women. The concept of basal-bolus insulin therapy (see Section: Insulin, pages 36–58) provides an ideal means of achieving good glucose control. Insulin pump therapy provides excellent control, but initiation of pump therapy must be accompanied by an intensive educational programme and close monitoring on the part of the whole team in terms of glucose monitoring and insulin management.[114,129]

Insulin therapies

Basal isophane (NPH) insulin provides the basis for good control with injections required in the morning and again at bedtime to provide adequate basal levels. Soluble (regular) insulin is then given prior to each meal and before any large snacks. The insulin analogues, insulin lispro and insulin aspart are very effective in controlling postprandial glucose and are of particular advantage in women who cannot predict the quantity of food that they will eat at any specific meal.[129–133]

The long-acting insulin analogue, insulin glargine, has not been assessed during pregnancy, and thus at this stage is not recommended as a basal insulin.

Management during delivery

There are many different programmes designed to manage the diabetic woman during delivery. The goal is to maintain tight glycaemic control until the baby is delivered, as elevated foetal blood glucose levels during the delivery time can lead to an excessive production of insulin from the foetal pancreas and the baby may then be born in a hypoglycaemic state. In many instances, the woman is asked not to eat or drink once labour has commenced and thus fluids, glucose, and insulin must be managed accordingly. An example of such a delivery routine is shown in Table 45.

Table 45. Management during delivery (assuming the patient is fasting during labour)

1. On admission to the labour suite, commence 2-hour glucose monitoring

2. Commence intravenous glucose (5%) at 100 ml/hour

3. Maintain plasma glucose below 6.5 mmol/l

4. If glucose is above 6.5 mmol/l, check 1 hour later and if still above 6.5 mmol/l commence iv insulin

5. Commence iv soluble/analogue insulin at 0.5 units per hour

6. Commence hourly self-glucose monitoring

7. Double hourly rate of iv insulin as required, until glucose maintained below 6.5 mmol/l. Continue to adjust iv insulin rate as required

8. As baby and placenta are delivered, discontinue iv insulin, but maintain iv dextrose infusion

9. Continue 2 hourly monitoring following delivery watching specifically for hypoglycaemia

10. As the patient may remain very sensitive to insulin in the postpartum period, do not commence insulin until plasma glucose levels are clearly rising

11. Commence insulin at low doses and titrate upwards according to levels of plasma glucose

At the completion of every pregnancy, it is important to sit down with the new mother to discuss issues of diabetes management. While the family's focus will now be on the new baby, it is important to emphasize with the patient, the need for ongoing diabetes care. Equally important, are the issues of the timing of potential further pregnancies and contraception.

After the intensive management of the diabetic pregnancy it is important to allow the mother to relax, but at the same time establish certain guidelines and parameters for diabetes control. A follow-up appointment for management of diabetes, including appropriate blood work, should be established within 3 months of the completion of the pregnancy.

Gestational diabetes

Gestational diabetes mellitus (GDM) can be defined as "glucose intolerance with onset of first recognition during pregnancy".[134] GDM may in fact be an expression of the impaired glucose tolerance state or an early presentation of Type 2 diabetes. The child of a woman with GDM is at increased risk for macrosomia, perinatal morbidity, foetal and maternal birth trauma and neonatal hypoglycaemia.[135–138]

The diagnosis of GDM remains controversial with many different standards having been established throughout the world.[139] Major studies such as the International Hyperglycemia and Adverse Pregnancy Outcome (HAPO) study may provide more long-term information. In general, a glucose load using the 75 g tolerance test is used to assess carbohydrate tolerance and it is now recommended that all pregnant women be

Table 46. Predictive risk factors for the presence of gestational diabetes
• family history of Type 2 diabetes
• obesity
• ethnic origin
• previous gestational diabetes
• previous diagnosis of IGT

Table 47. Diagnostic criteria for gestational diabetes		
1. Using a fasting 75 g glucose load		
Timing of glucose test	**Glucose mmol/l**	**GDM criteria**
Fasting plasma glucose	>5.3	2 values are met
One hour postprandial	≥ 10.6	or exceeded
Two hour postprandial	≥ 8.9	
2. Using 50 g glucose load, given at anytime of the day		
Timing of glucose test	**Glucose mmol/l**	**GDM criteria**
One hour postprandial	≥ 10.3	Confirmed GDM
One hour postprandial	7.8–10.3	75 g OGTT recommended

screened between 24 and 28 weeks of gestation. Frequently, a 50 g glucose tolerance test is utilized as the screening test.

The presence of several risk factors may predict the presence of GDM (Table 46). Typical diagnostic criteria for GDM are shown in Table 47.

Management of GDM
Nutritional therapy
Nutritional therapy is the basis of management of GDM and it is important to individualize the diet with each patient. In many patients, obesity has been a problem prior to the commencement of the pregnancy and once again it is not appropriate to make a major reduction in calories. Nevertheless, a readjustment of calories will frequently lead to a decrease in postprandial glucose.[140–142]

Physical activity is an important adjunct to the diet and again may assist in decreasing postprandial glucose.[143]

Glucose monitoring
Self-glucose monitoring in both the preprandial and postprandial periods will provide an excellent indication of glucose control.[123] The goals are outlined in Table 43.

Insulin therapy

If target glucose levels have not been reached, insulin therapy should be initiated. Initially basal insulins, in conjunction with an appropriate diet, may be sufficient to achieve glucose targets. If glucose values are rising, intensive insulin therapy will be required.[133,144] The goal always, is to reach pre- and postprandial glucose targets throughout the pregnancy.

Initially, isophane insulin may be required at either breakfast or bedtime, or at both times, depending on the time of day when hyperglycaemia has been noted. Soluble insulin or fast-acting analogue insulin, may be required prior to each meal to achieve ideal postprandial glucose targets.

Postpartum assessment

This is a most important aspect of the management of the patient with GDM. Once the baby has been delivered, a discussion should take place with the mother to review her long-term health. A sensible weight goal should be established for the months following the pregnancy, as well as practical dietary and exercise routines. An assessment of carbohydrate tolerance should be made within 3 months of the delivery to ensure that the patient has returned to a normal metabolic state.

There is an increased risk of developing Type 2 diabetes following GDM and thus the patient needs to be advised of appropriate glucose testing, to be performed on a routine basis during regular medical examinations.

Frequently Asked Questions

Why is there a massive explosion in the numbers of people being diagnosed with Type 2 diabetes in the world?

Increasing levels of obesity and the increasingly sedentary lifestyle of many people in the world are the main factors.

When should physicians perform an oral glucose tolerance test (OGTT) to diagnose diabetes?

The diagnosis of Type 2 diabetes is usually straightforward. A person presents with symptoms suggestive of diabetes, such as thirst, polyuria and tiredness, and has a random blood glucose value above 11.1 mmol/l, which confirms the diagnosis.

In situations where people present with symptoms and random blood glucose is not diagnostic, a fasting blood glucose level above 7 mmol/l confirms the diagnosis.

An OGTT is needed when a person with symptoms has a fasting glucose result in the range 6–7 mmol/l (impaired fasting glucose), or where an asymptomatic individual has two fasting glucose values in the IFG range.

Should we carry out population screening of asymptomatic individuals for Type 2 diabetes?

In the UK it is felt that the jury is still out! More research is thought to be needed on its cost-effectiveness in different populations. Opportunistic screening of high-risk populations, e.g. those with known cardiovascular disease, hypertension, those with a BMI above 30, etc, should be done.

How can individuals with diabetes be empowered to look after themselves?

People need to be given the information they need to enable them to understand and self-manage their diabetes. Good education, beginning at diagnosis, and continuing at each consultation is very important.

The person with diabetes needs to feel able to ask questions. A consultation style that facilitates this might include questions such as "What is the most difficult thing for you at the moment in looking after your diabetes?"

Should people with diabetes blood glucose monitor?

Everyone who is on insulin, whether they have Type 1 or Type 2 diabetes, should be blood glucose monitoring. This will enable them to vary their insulin dose in response to the varying levels of activity and food they have during the week. The frequency of monitoring will vary for each person, and needs to reflect the week by week variation in their life events.

There is a degree of disagreement as to whether people with Type 2 diabetes who are controlled on tablets and/or diet need to be encouraged to blood glucose monitor. Those against it argue that it can be quite expensive to health budgets, and there is only a little evidence that it improves overall glycaemic control. Outcomes in Type 2 diabetes are predicated on HbA_{1c} values which can be determined every 3 months, and people with Type 2 diabetes cannot alter the number of tablets they take each day depending on their blood glucose monitoring.

Those in favour of blood glucose monitoring in Type 2 diabetes argue that it allows the individual to quickly understand the relationship of blood glucose to eating particular foods and taking exercise, and is therefore a tremendous benefit in empowering the person with diabetes.

One course of action is to ensure that everyone on insulin is taught and has the equipment to blood glucose monitor. Once stabilized they are encouraged to monitor when and if they feel it will help them to control their diabetes optimally.

The opportunity to learn about blood glucose monitoring should be offered to all with Type 2 diabetes not on insulin, but don't push it if they don't want to.

Does this 45-year-old person newly diagnosed with diabetes have Type 1 or Type 2 diabetes?

Type 1 diabetes can occur at any age, although it is usually in childhood or adolescence. Sometimes people present with a short history and quite pronounced symptoms, and perhaps have a blood glucose at diagnosis of say 25 mmol/l and greater. Do they have Type 1 and should they have insulin straight away?

Other factors suggestive of Type 1 are a thin patient with a history of weight loss and ketonuria. Factors suggestive of Type 2 are obesity and high sugar intake.

Sometimes in a thin symptomatic person without ketonuria it is not completely clear.

One course of action is to treat them initially as Type 2 and give lifestyle advice education and use a sulphonylurea such as gliclazide. Then see them every 2 weeks and titrate the dose up as necessary using fasting blood glucose as the measure of glycaemia, always remembering that they may need to go on insulin if the symptoms and glycaemia are not adequately controlled. If they require insulin therapy within 1 year of diagnosis they will be retrospectively labelled as having Type 1 diabetes.

How can the subject of erectile dysfunction (ED) be brought up in a consultation?

Many people with diabetes feel very embarrassed about discussing ED with their healthcare team, and we may feel embarrassed asking them. Questions that can help include "Some men with diabetes develop problems with erections, I wondered if you were having any difficulties?"

Why do I have to take so many tablets to manage my diabetes – I would prefer to keep on just diet and exercise for treatment?

Diabetes is a progressive disease and blood sugars will continue to rise year after year. Thus, it is important that we treat the high sugar quickly to stop the glucose levels from getting too high and this will often require two or even three medications.

I am taking tablets for my diabetes. Why do I have to take extra tablets for high blood pressure and cholesterol?

Diabetes is a complex disease with three abnormalities often being present which can contribute to heart disease. The three abnormalities include high sugars, high blood pressure and abnormal lipids (high cholesterol). Thus, it is important to treat all three abnormalities to help reduce the risk of heart disease in the future.

I know my blood sugars are high, but I am on tablets so why do I have to take insulin?

After many years of diabetes, even tablets will not control blood sugar, as the pancreas is unable to make enough insulin. Thus, even a small amount of insulin can help correct the high blood sugar and allow the tablets to work even better.

I am very scared of taking insulin. Doesn't it make my blood sugars go too low?

We now have techniques to give insulin using a simple device called the insulin pen. Often insulin is only required at night-time but if it is required during the day, new types of insulin can be used that will reduce the risk of low blood sugars. Once using insulin you will be pleased how well controlled your diabetes can be without any major increase in risk to yourself.

What is the best way to treat a low blood sugar – I usually use a chocolate bar?

It is best to use a glucose that is rapidly absorbed and the most convenient way to do this is by taking glucose tablets. If these are not available then a fruit juice such as orange juice or apple juice should be taken to correct the low blood sugar.

I often find my morning blood sugar is high even though it was at a good level when I went to bed. Why is this?

Overnight, the body can produce excess glucose causing the blood sugar to rise. This can often be corrected by using tablets that lower the sugar levels but if sugars remain too high, a small dose of insulin taken at bedtime can solve the problem.

I have been told that I will have terrible problems from my diabetes – I could lose my sight; my kidneys could fail and I could even lose a leg. Is this true?

We now know that if all the abnormalities of diabetes, elevated blood sugar, elevated blood pressure and elevated cholesterol levels are all corrected, the risks to you of developing serious vascular diseases as you have described, will be greatly reduced and may in some people be eliminated.

As a woman, I would like to have children but have been told that I can't because I have diabetes. Is this true?

Women with diabetes are definitely able to have a successful pregnancy. The key will be excellent glucose control before you conceive and during the pregnancy. With good control of diabetes there is not a lot of difference between a woman with diabetes or a woman without diabetes when having children, apart from the need for close supervision and management for the pregnant woman with diabetes.

I am pregnant with my first child and have been told that I'll have to deliver my baby, maybe by caesarian section, many weeks before the due date, to protect the baby because of my diabetes. Is this true?

If your diabetes has been under good control and there are no obstetric concerns, there is no reason why you will not be able to deliver your baby on the due date and without the need for the caesarean section.

After struggling so hard to lose weight, now that my diabetes is controlled, I am actually gaining weight. Why?

Most of the medications that help control diabetes will cause weight gain, especially insulin. When considering two bad situations – weight gain or higher blood sugars, it is the need to lower the sugar levels that becomes the most important to achieve. Sadly, this will often result in a weight gain of 2–4 kg (4–7 lbs). With careful attention to diet and a good exercise programme, this weight gain can be kept to a minimum.

References

1. Alberti KGMM, Zimmet PZ, for the WHO consultation. Definition, Diagnosis and Classification of Diabetes Mellitus and its Complications. Part 1: Diagnosis and Classification of Diabetes Mellitus. Provisional Report of a WHO consultation. *Diabetic Medicine* 1998; **15**: 539–553.

2. British Diabetic Association (now Diabetes UK). *New Diagnostic Criteria for Diabetes*. London UK: 30 April 2000.

3. Narayan KM, Imperatore G, Benjamin SM *et al*. Targetting people with pre-diabetes (editorial). *BMJ* 2002; **325**: 965.

4. Alberti KG. Impaired glucose tolerance: what are the clinical implications. *Diabetes Res Clin Pract* 1998; **40** (suppl): 53–58.

5. Tuomilehto JLJ, Eriksson JG, Valle TT *et al*. Prevention of Type 2 diabetes mellitus by changes in lifestyle among subjects with impaired glucose tolerance. *New Engl J Med* 2001; **344**: 1343–1392.

6. The Diabetes Prevention Programme Research Group. Reduction in the incidence of Type 2 diabetes with lifestyle intervention or metformin. *New Engl J Med* 2002; **346**: 393–403.

7. Chiasson J-L, Josse RG, Gomis R *et al*. Acarbose for prevention of type 2 diabetes mellitus: the STOP_NIDDM randomised trial. *Lancet* 2002; **359**: 2072–2077.

8. Sjostrom L, Torgerson JS, Hauptman J *et al*. XENDOS (XENical in the prevention of diabetes in obese subjects): a landmark study. Abstract presented at 9th Int Congress on Obesity. San Paulo, Brazil: 24–29 August 2002.

9. Singh B, Prescott J, Guy R *et al*. Effectiveness of poster campaign on the awareness of diabetes. *BMJ* 1994; **308**: 632–636.

10. Feltblower RG, McKinney HJ, Bodansky HJ. Diabetes in children in Yorkshire. *Diabetalogia* 2000; **43**: 381–389.

11. Diabetes Prevention Trial-Type 1 (DPT-1) Study Group. Effects of insulin in relatives of patients with Type 1 diabetes mellitus. *New Engl J Med* 2002; **346**: 1685–1691.

12. Phillips JC, Scheen AJ. Study of the prevention of Type 1 diabetes with nicotinamide (ENDIT study): positive lessons from a negative clinical trial. *Rev Med Liege* 2002; **57**: 672–675.

13. International Diabetes Federation (IDF). *Diabetes Atlas 2000*. Brussels, Belgium: July 2000.

14. Gadsby R. Epidemiology of Diabetes. *Advanced Drug Delivery System Reviews* 2002; **54**: 1165–1172.

15. Rosenbloom JR, Joe JR, Young RS *et al*. Emerging epidemic of Type 2 diabetes in youth. *Diabetes Care* 1999; **22**: 345–354.

16. Lawrence JM, Bennett P, Young A *et al*. Screening for diabetes in general practice: cross sectional study. *BMJ* 2001; **323**: 548–551.

17. Leiter LA *et al*. Diabetes Screening in Canada (DIASCAN) Study: prevalence of undiagnosed diabetes and glucose intolerance in family physician offices. *Diabetes Care* 2001; **24**(6): 1038–43.

18. Reaven GM. Banting Lecture. Role of insulin resistance in human disease. *Diabetes* 1988; **37**: 1595–1607.

19. Department of Health. *National Service Framework for Diabetes: Standards*. London: Department of Health, 2001.

20. Kanters SD, Banga JD, Stolk RP *et al*. Incidence and determinants of mortality and cardiovascular events in diabetes mellitus: a meta-analysis. *Vasc Med* 1999; **4**: 67–75.

21. Dawson KG *et al*. The economic cost of diabetes in Canada, 1998. *Diabetes Care* 2002; **25**(8): 1303–07.

22. Renders CM, Valk GD, Griffen S *et al*. Intervention to improve the management of diabetes in primary care, outpatient and community settings. *Diabetes Care* 2001; **24**: 1821–1833.

23. Griffen S. Diabetes care in general practice: meta-analysis of randomised controlled trials. *BMJ* 1998; **317**: 390–395.

24. Griffen S, Williams R. Delivering care to the population. In: Williams R, Herman JW, Kinmonth A-L *et al*, editors. *The Evidence Base for Diabetes Care*. Chichester: Wiley, 2002; chapter 32.

25. Day JL, Metacalfe J, Johnson P. Benefits provided by an integrated education and clinical diabetes centre: a follow up study. *Diabetic Medicine* 1992; **9**: 855–859.

26. Jaber LA, Halapy H, Fernet M *et al*. Evaluation of a pharmaceutical care model on diabetes management. *Ann Pharmacother* 1996; **30**: 238–243.

27. Peters AL, Davidson MB. Application of a diabetes managed care

program. The feasibility of using nurses and a computer system to provide effective care. *Diabetes Care* 1998; **21**: 1037–1043.

28. Aubert RE, Herman WH, Waters J *et al.* Nurse case management to improve glycaemic control in diabetic patients in a health maintenance organization. *Ann Intern Med* 1998; **129**: 605–612.

29. IDF Consultative Section on Diabetes Education. *International Consensus Standards of Practice for Diabetes Education.* London: Class Publishing, 1997.

30. Education Study Group of EASD. Survival Kit. A Document for health care providers and patients: working party report. *Diabetic Medicine* 1995; **12**: 1022–1043.

31. SIGN Executive. *SIGN Guideline 55 – Management of Diabetes.* Edinburgh, Scotland: 2001. (www.sign.ac.uk)

32. Estabrooks PA, Glasgow RE, Dzewaltowski DA. Physical activity promotion through primary care. *JAMA* 2003; **289**: 2913–2916.

33. MacKinnon M. *Providing Diabetes Care in General Practice.* 4th Edition. London: Class Publishing, 2002.

34. Bott U, Bott S, Hemmann D *et al.* Evaluation of a holistic treatment and teaching programme for patients with Type 1 diabetes who failed to achieve their goals under intensified insulin therapy. *Diabetic Medicine* 2000; **17**: 635–643.

35. DAPHNE study group. Training in flexible, intensive insulin management to enable dietary freedom in people with type 1 diabetes: dose adjustment for normal eating (DAFNE) randomised controlled trial. *BMJ* 2002; **325**: 746–751.

36. Diabetes Control and Complications Trial Research Group. The effect of intensive treatment of diabetes on the development and progression of long term complications in insulin dependent diabetes mellitus. *New Engl J Med* 1993; **329**: 977–986.

37. UKPDS Group. Effect of intensive blood glucose control with sulphonylureas or insulin compared with conventional treatment and risk of complications in patients with type 2 diabetes (UKPDS 33). *Lancet* 1998; **352**: 837–853.

38. Stratton IM, Adler AI, Neil HA *et al.* Association of glycaemia with macrovascular and microvascular complications in type 2 diabetes UKPDS 35. *BMJ* 2000; **321**: 405–411.

39. Chatterjee M, Scobie I. The pathogenesis of type 2 diabetes mellitus. *Practical Diabetes International* 2002; **19**(8): 255–257.

40. Haffner S. The importance of hyperglycemia in the nonfasting state to the development of cardiovascular disease. *Endocr Rev* 1998; **19**: 583–592.

41. Hanefeld M, Temelkova-Kurktschiev T. The postprandial state and the risk of atherosclerosis. *Diabet Med* 1997; **14**(Suppl 3): S6–S11.

42. Fonseca V *et al*. Effect of metformin and rosiglitazone combination therapy in patients with type 2 diabetes mellitus: a randomized controlled trial. *JAMA* 2000; **283**(13): 1695–1702.

43. Buchanan TA *et al*. Preservation of pancreatic beta-cell function and prevention of type 2 diabetes by pharmacological treatment of insulin resistance in high-risk hispanic women. *Diabetes* 2002; **51**(9): 2796–2803.

44. Drouin P. Diamicron MR once daily is effective and well tolerated in type 2 diabetes: a double-blind, randomized, multinational study. *J Diabetes Complications* 2000; **14**(4): 185–191.

45. Campbell RK. Glimepiride: role of a new sulfonylurea in the treatment of type 2 diabetes mellitus. *Ann Pharmacother* 1998; **32**(10): 1044–1052.

46. Chiasson JL *et al*. The efficacy of acarbose in the treatment of patients with non-insulin-dependent diabetes mellitus. A multicenter controlled clinical trial. *Ann Intern Med* 1994; **121**(12): 928–935.

47. Klein R, Klein BEK, Moss SE *et al*. The Wisconsin Epidemiological Study of Diabetic Retinopathy 111. Prevalence and risk of diabetic retinopathy when age at diagnosis is 30 years or more. *Arch Opthalmol* 1984; **102**: 527–532.

48. NICE Inherited Clinical Guidance. *Management of Type 2 Diabetes: Retinopathy – Screening and Early Management.* London: NICE, 2002.

49. United Kingdom Prospective Diabetes Study Group. Tight blood pressure control and risk of macrovascular and microvascular complications in type 2 diabetes (UKPDS 38). *BMJ* 1998; **317**: 703–713.

50. Kohner E. Commentary: Treatment of diabetic retinopathy. *BMJ* 2003; **326**: 1024–1025.

51. Chaturvedi N, Sjolie A, Styephenson JM and the EUCLID study group. Effect of lisinopril on progression of retinopathy in normotensive people with type 1 diabetes. *Lancet* 1998; **351**: 28–31.

52. Parving G, Hommel E, Mathiesen E *et al.* Prevalence of microalbuminuria, arterial hypertension, and neuropathy in patients with insulin dependant diabetes mellitus. *BMJ* 1988; **296**: 156–160.

53. Hutchinson A, McIntosh A, Feder G *et al. Clinical Guidelines and Evidence Review Type 2 Diabetes – Prevention & Management of Foot Problems.* London: RCGP, 2000.

54. The EUCLID Study Group. Randomised placebo controlled trial of lisinopril in normotensive patients with insulin dependant diabetes mellitus and normoalbuminuria or microalbuminuria. *Lancet* 1997; **349**: 1787–1792.

55. Heart Outcomes Prevention Evaluation (HOPE) Study Investigators. Effects of ramipril on cardiovascular and microvascular outcomes in people with diabetes mellitus: the results of the HOPE study and the MICRO-HOPE substudy. *Lancet* 2000; **355**: 2593–2599.

56. Parving HH, Lehnert H, Brocher-Mortensen J *et al.* The effect of irbesartan on the development of diabetic nephropathy in patients with type 2 diabetes. *New Engl J Med* 2001; **345**: 870–878.

57. Pedrini MT, Levey AS, Lau J *et al.* The effect of dietary protein restriction on the progression of diabetic and non diabetic renal disease: a meta-analysis. *Ann Int Med* 1996; **124**: 627–632.

58. Boulton AJ. The pathway to ulceration: aetiopathogenesis. In: Boulton A, Connor H, Cavanagh P, editors. *The Foot in Diabetes.* Third edition. Chichester: John Wiley and Sons, 2000; Chapter 3.

59. Ziegler D. Diagnosis and management of diabetic peripheral neuropathy. *Diabetic Medicine* 1996; **13**: S34–S38.

60. Gadsby R, McInnes A. The "at risk foot": the role of the primary care team in acheiving St Vincent targets for reducing amputation. *Diabetic Medicine* 1998; **15** (Suppl 3): S61–S64.

61. Kumar S, Fernando D, Veves A *et al.* Semmes-Weinstein monofilaments, a simple device for identifying diabetes patients at risk of foot ulceration. *Diabetes Res Clin Pract* 1991; **13**: 63–68.

62. Boulton A, Gries F, Jervell J. Guidelines for the diagnosis and outpatient management of diabetic peripheral neuropathy. *Diabetic Medicine* 1998; **15**: 508–514.

63. Edmonds M, Blundell M, Morris H *et al.* The diabetic foot: impact of foot advice. *Quart J Med* 1986; **232**: 763–771.

64. Lakin MM, Montague DK, Vanderbrig Medendorp S *et al.* Intracavernous injection therapy: analysis of results and complications. *J Urology* 1990; **143**: 1138–1141.

65. Spollett GR. Assessment and management of erectile dysfunction in men with diabetes. *Diabetes Educator* 1999; **25**: 65–73.

66. Rendell MS, Rajfer J, Wicker P *et al* for the Sildenafil Diabetes Study Group. Sildenafil for treatment of erectile dysfunction in men with diabetes: a randomised controlled study. *JAMA* 1999; **281**: 421–426.

67. Genest J *et al.* Recommendations for the management of dyslipidemia and the prevention of cardiovascular disease: 2003 update. *Can Med Assoc J* 2003; **168**(9): online-1–online-10.

68. Timar O, Sestier F, Levy E. Metabolic syndrome X: a review. *Can J Cardiol* 2000; **16**(6): 779–789.

69. Fernandez-Real JM, Ricart W. Insulin resistance and chronic cardiovascular inflammatory syndrome. *Endocr Rev* 2003; **24**(3): 278–301.

70. Lemieux S, Despres JP. Metabolic complications of visceral obesity: contribution to the aetiology of type 2 diabetes and implications for prevention and treatment. *Diabete Metab* 1994; **20**(4): 375–393.

71. Reaven GM. Resistance to insulin-stimulated glucose uptake and hyperinsulinemia: role in non-insulin-dependent diabetes, high blood pressure, dyslipidemia and coronary heart disease. *Diabete & Metabolisme (Paris)* 1991; **17**: 78–86.

72. Zhao X *et al.* Simvastatin plus niacin protect against atherosclerosis progression and clinical events in coronary artery disease patients with metabolic syndrome. *J Am Coll Cardiol* 2002; **39**(5 Suppl A): 242.

73. Gokcel A *et al.* Effects of sibutramine in obese female subjects with type 2 diabetes and poor blood glucose control. *Diabetes Care* 2001; **24**(11): 1957–1960.

74. Hanefeld M, Sachse G. The effects of orlistat on body weight and glycaemic control in overweight patients with type 2 diabetes: a randomized, placebo-controlled trial. *Diabetes Obes Metab* 2002; **4**(6): 415–423.

75. Finer N. Pharmacotherapy of obesity. *Best Pract Res Clin Endocrinol Metab* 2002; **16**(4): 717–742.

76. Arauz-Pacheco C, Parrott MA, Raskin P. Treatment of hypertension in adults with diabetes. *Diabetes Care* 2003; **26**(Suppl 1): S80–S82.

77. Pyorala K *et al*. Cholesterol lowering with simvastatin improves prognosis of diabetic patients with coronary heart disease: a subgroup analysis of the Scandanavian Simvastatin Survival Study (4S). *Diabetes Care* 1997; **20**: 614–620.

78. MRC/BHF Heart Protection Study of cholesterol lowering with simvastatin in 20,536 high-risk individuals: a randomised placebo-controlled trial. *Lancet* 2002; **360**(9326): 7–22.

79. Sever PS *et al*. Prevention of coronary and stroke events with ator-vastatin in hypertensive patients who have average or lower-than-average cholesterol concentrations, in the Anglo-Scandinavian Cardiac Outcomes Trial—Lipid Lowering Arm (ASCOT-LLA): a multicentre randomised controlled trial. *Lancet* 2003; **361**(9364): 1149–1158.

80. Brenner BM *et al*. Effects of losartan on renal and cardiovascular outcomes in patients with type 2 diabetes and nephropathy. *New Engl J Med* 2001; **345**(12): 861–869.

81. Lewis EJ *et al*. Renoprotective effect of the angiotensin-receptor antagonist irbesartan in patients with nephropathy due to type 2 diabetes. *New Engl J Med* 2001; **345**(12): 851–860.

82. Kirpichnikov D, Winer N, Sowers JR. The use of ACE inhibitors on diabetic patients without renal disease. *Curr Diab Rep* 2002; **2**(1): 21–25.

83. Lewis EJ *et al*. The effect of angiotensin-converting-enzyme inhibi-tion on diabetic nephropathy. *New Engl J Med* 1993; **329**: 1456–1462.

84. Melbourne Diabetic Nephropathy Study Group. Comparison between perindopril and nifedipine in hypertensive and normotensive diabetic patients with microalbuminuria. *BMJ* 1991; **302**: 210–216.

85. Gaede P *et al*. Multifactorial intervention and cardiovascular disease in patients with type 2 diabetes. *N Engl J Med* 2003; **348**(5): 383–93.

86. Colwell JA. Aspirin therapy in diabetes. *Diabetes Care* 2003; **26**(Suppl 1): S87–S88.

87. Cryer PE. Banting Lecture. Hypoglycemia: the limiting factor in the management of IDDM. *Diabetes* 1994; **43**(11): 1378–1389.

88. Yale JF *et al*. 2001 Canadian Diabetes Association Clinical Practice Guidelines for the Prevention and Management of Hypoglycemia in Diabetes. *Canadian J Diagnosis* 2002; **26**: 22–25.

89. Bolli G *et al*. Abnormal glucose counterregulation in insulin-dependent diabetes mellitus. Interaction of anti-insulin antibodies and

impaired glucagon and epinephrine secretion. *Diabetes* 1983; **32**(2): 134–141.

90. Dagogo-Jack S, Fanelli CG, Cryer PE. Durable reversal of hypo-glycemia unawareness in type 1 diabetes. *Diabetes Care* 1999; **22**(5): 866–867.

91. Liu D, McManus RM, Ryan EA. Improved counter-regulatory hormonal and symptomatic responses to hypoglycemia in patients with insulin-dependent diabetes mellitus after 3 months of less strict glycemic control. *Clin Invest Med* 1996; **19**(2): 71–82.

92. Effects of intensive diabetes therapy on neuropsychological function in adults in the Diabetes Control and Complications Trial. *Ann Intern Med* 1996; **124**(4): 379–388.

93. Ryan CM *et al*. Cognitive dysfunction in adults with type 1 (insulin-dependent) diabetes mellitus of long duration: effects of recurrent hypo-glycaemia and other chronic complications. *Diabetologia* 1993; **36**(4): 329–334.

94. Northam EA *et al*. Neuropsychological complications of IDDM in children 2 years after disease onset. *Diabetes Care* 1998; **21**(3): 379–384.

95. Clarke WL *et al*. The relationship between nonroutine use of insulin, food, and exercise and the occurrence of hypoglycemia in adults with IDDM and varying degrees of hypoglycemic awareness and metabolic control. *Diabetes Educ* 1997; **23**(1): 55–58.

96. MacLeod KM, Gold AE, Frier BM. A comparative study of respons-es to acute hypoglycaemia induced by human and porcine insulins in patients with Type 1 diabetes. *Diabet Med* 1996; **13**(4): 346–357.

97. Colagiuri S, Miller JJ, Petocz P. Double-blind crossover comparison of human and porcine insulins in patients reporting lack of hypogly-caemia awareness. *Lancet* 1992; **339**(8807): 1432–1435.

98. Berger W *et al*. [The relatively frequent incidence of severe sulfony-lurea-induced hypoglycemia in the last 25 years in Switzerland. Results of 2 surveys in Switzerland in 1969 and 1984]. *Schweiz Med Wochenschr* 1986; **116**(5): 145–151.

99. Tessier D *et al*. Glibenclamide vs gliclazide in type 2 diabetes of the elderly. *Diabet Med* 1994; **11**(10): 974–980.

100. Damsbo P *et al*. A double-blind randomized comparison of meal-related glycemic control by repaglinide and glyburide in well-controlled type 2 diabetic patients. *Diabetes Care* 1999; **22**(5): 789–794.

101. DeFronzo RA, Goodman AM. Efficacy of metformin in patients with non-insulin-dependent diabetes mellitus. The Multicenter Metformin Study Group. *New Engl J Med* 1995; **333**(9): 541–549.

102. Slama G *et al*. The search for an optimized treatment of hypoglycemia. Carbohydrates in tablets, solution, or gel for the correction of insulin reactions. *Arch Intern Med* 1990; **150**(3): 589–593.

103. Cryer PE, Fisher JN, Shamoon H. Hypoglycemia. *Diabetes Care* 1994; **17**(7): 734–755.

104. Palatnick W, Meatherall RC, Tenenbein M. Clinical spectrum of sulfonylurea overdose and experience with diazoxide therapy. *Arch Intern Med* 1991; **151**(9): 1859–1862.

105. Chiasson JL *et al*. Diagnosis and treatment of diabetic ketoacidosis and the hyperglycemic hyperosmolar state. *CMAJ* 2003; **168**(7): 859–866.

106. MacIsaac RJ *et al*. Influence of age on the presentation and outcome of acidotic and hyperosmolar diabetic emergencies. *Intern Med J* 2002; **32**(8): 379–385.

107. Wiggam MI *et al*. Treatment of diabetic ketoacidosis using normalization of blood 3-hydroxybutyrate concentration as the endpoint of emergency management. A randomized controlled study. *Diabetes Care* 1997; **20**(9): 1347–1352.

108. Gonzalez-Campoy JM, Robertson RP. Diabetic ketoacidosis and hyperosmolar nonketotic state: gaining control over extreme hyperglycemic complications. *Postgrad Med* 1996; **99**(6): 143–152.

109. Kitabchi AE *et al*. Hyperglycemic crises in patients with diabetes mellitus. *Diabetes Care* 2003; **26**(Suppl 1): S109–S117.

110. Schaefer-Graf UM *et al*. Patterns of congenital anomalies and relationship to initial maternal fasting glucose levels in pregnancies complicated by type 2 and gestational diabetes. *Am J Obstet Gynecol* 2000; **182**(2): 313–320.

111. Suhonen L, Hiilesmaa V, Teramo K. Glycaemic control during early pregnancy and fetal malformations in women with type I diabetes mellitus. *Diabetologia* 2000; **43**(1): 79–82.

112. Farrell T, Neale L, Cundy T. Congenital anomalies in the offspring of women with type 1, type 2 and gestational diabetes. *Diabet Med* 2002; **19**(4): 322–326.

113. McElvy SS *et al*. A focused preconceptional and early pregnancy program in women with type 1 diabetes reduces perinatal mortality and malformation rates to general population levels. *J Matern Fetal Med* 2000; **9**(1): 14–20.

114. Howorka K *et al*. Normalization of pregnancy outcome in pregestational diabetes through functional insulin treatment and modular out-patient education adapted for pregnancy. *Diabet Med* 2001; **18**(12): 965–972.

115. Kitzmiller JL *et al*. Preconception care of diabetes: glycemic control prevents congenital anomalies. *JAMA* 1991; **265**: 731–736.

116. Preconception care of women with diabetes. *Diabetes Care* 2003; **26**(Suppl 1): S91–S93.

117. Kitzmiller JL *et al*. Pre-conception care of diabetes, congenital malformations, and spontaneous abortions. *Diabetes Care* 1996; **19**(5): 514–541.

118. Cundy T *et al*. Perinatal mortality in Type 2 diabetes mellitus. *Diabet Med* 2000; **17**(1): 33–39.

119. Feig DS, Palda VA. Type 2 diabetes in pregnancy: a growing concern. *Lancet* 2002; **359**(9318): 1690–1692.

120. Kitzmiller JL, Combs CA. Diabetic nephropathy and pregnancy. *Obstet Gynecol Clin North Am* 1996; **23**(1): 173–203.

121. Schaefer UM *et al*. Congenital malformations in offspring of women with hyperglycemia first detected during pregnancy. *Am J Obstet Gynecol* 1997; **177**(5): 1165–1171.

122. Bar J *et al*. Pregnancy outcome in patients with insulin dependent diabetes mellitus and diabetic nephropathy treated with ACE inhibitors before pregnancy. *J Pediatr Endocrinol Metab* 1999; **12**(5): 659–665.

123. Combs CA *et al*. Relationship of fetal macrosomia to maternal postprandial glucose control during pregnancy. *Diabetes Care* 1992; **15**(10): 1251–1257.

124. Evidence-based nutrition principles and recommendations for the treatment and prevention of diabetes and related complications. *Diabetes Care* 2002; **25**(1): 202–212.

125. Mann J *et al*. Evidence-based nutritional recommendations for the treatment and prevention of diabetes and related complications: a European perspective. *Diabetes Care* 2002; **25**(7): 1256–1258.

126. Jovanovic L. Medical nutritional therapy in pregnant women with pregestational diabetes mellitus. *J Matern Fetal Med* 2000; **9**(1): 21–28.

127. Montaner P, Dominguez R, Corcoy R. Self-monitored blood glucose in pregnant women without gestational diabetes mellitus. *Diabetes Care* 2002; **25**(11): 2104–2105.

128. Diamond MP *et al*. Impairment of counterregulatory hormone responses to hypoglycemia in pregnant women with insulin-dependent diabetes mellitus. *Am J Obstet Gynecol* 1992; **166**(1): 70–77.

129. Burkart W, Hanker JP, Schneider HP. Complications and fetal outcome in diabetic pregnancy. Intensified conventional versus insulin pump therapy. *Gynecol Obstet Invest* 1988; **26**(2): 104–112.

130. Masson EA *et al*. Pregnancy outcome in Type 1 diabetes mellitus treated with insulin lispro (Humalog). *Diabet Med* 2003; **20**(1): 46–50.

131. Pettitt DJ *et al*. Comparison of an insulin analog, insulin aspart, and regular human insulin with no insulin in gestational diabetes mellitus. *Diabetes Care* 2003; **26**(1): 183–186.

132. Jovanovic L *et al*. Metabolic and immunologic effects of insulin lispro in gestational diabetes. *Diabetes Care* 1999; **22**(9): 1422–1427.

133. Nachum Z *et al*. Twice daily versus four times daily insulin dose regimens for diabetes in pregnancy: randomised controlled trial. *BMJ* 1999; **319**(7219): 1223–1227.

134. Metzger BE, Coustan DR. Summary and recommendations of the Fourth International Workshop-Conference on Gestational Diabetes Mellitus. The Organizing Committee. *Diabetes Care* 1998; **21**(Suppl 2): B161–B167.

135. Berger H *et al*. Screening for gestational diabetes mellitus. *J Obstet Gynaecol Can* 2002; **24**(11): 894–912.

136. Griffin ME *et al*. Universal vs. risk factor-based screening for gestational diabetes mellitus: detection rates, gestation at diagnosis and outcome. *Diabet Med* 2000; **17**(1): 26–32.

137. Schaefer-Graf UM *et al*. Determinants of fetal growth at different periods of pregnancies complicated by gestational diabetes mellitus or impaired glucose tolerance. *Diabetes Care* 2003; **26**(1): 193–198.

138. Adams KM *et al*. Sequelae of unrecognized gestational diabetes. *Am J Obstet Gynecol* 1998; **178**(6): 1321–1332.

139. Metzger BE. 1990 overview of GDM. Accomplishments of the last decade—challenges for the future. *Diabetes* 1991; **40**(Suppl 2): 1-2.

140. Jovanovic L, Pettitt DJ. Gestational diabetes mellitus. *JAMA* 2001; **286**(20): 2516–2518.

141. Dornhorst A, Frost G. The principles of dietary management of gestational diabetes: reflection on current evidence. *J Hum Nutr Diet* 2002; **15**(2): 145–156.

142. Jensen DM *et al*. Clinical impact of mild carbohydrate intolerance in pregnancy: a study of 2904 nondiabetic Danish women with risk factors for gestational diabetes mellitus. *Am J Obstet Gynecol* 2001; **185**(2): 413–419.

143. Avery MD, Walker AJ. Acute effect of exercise on blood glucose and insulin levels in women with gestational diabetes. *J Matern Fetal Med* 2001; **10**(1): 52–58.

144. Hadden DR. When and how to start insulin treatment in gestational diabetes: a UK perspective. *Diabet Med* 2001; **18**(12): 960–964.

Further Reading on Insulin

Bode BW, Strange P. Efficacy, safety, and pump compatibility of insulin aspart used in continuous subcutaneous insulin infusion therapy in patients with type 1 diabetes. *Diabetes Care* 2001; **24**(1): 69–72.

Boehm BO *et al*. Premixed insulin aspart 30 vs. premixed human insulin 30/70 twice daily: a randomized trial in Type 1 and Type 2 diabetic patients. *Diabet Med* 2002; **19**(5): 393–399.

Bolli GB *et al*. Insulin analogues and their potential in the management of diabetes mellitus. *Diabetologia* 1999; **42**(10): 1151–1167.

DeVries JH *et al*. A randomized trial of insulin aspart with intensified basal NPH insulin supplementation in people with Type 1 diabetes. *Diabet Med* 2003; **20**(4): 312–318.

Home PD, Ashwell SG. An overview of insulin glargine. *Diabetes Metab Res Rev* 2002; **18**(Suppl 3): S57-S63.

Home PD, Lindholm A, Riis A. Insulin aspart vs. human insulin in the management of long-term blood glucose control in Type 1 diabetes mellitus: a randomized controlled trial. *Diabet Med* 2000; **17**(11): 762–770.

Lalli C *et al*. Long-term intensive treatment of type 1 diabetes with the short-acting insulin analog lispro in variable combination with NPH insulin at mealtime. *Diabetes Care* 1999; **22**(3): 468–477.

Malone JK *et al*. Improved postprandial glycemic control with Humalog Mix75/25 after a standard test meal in patients with type 2 diabetes mellitus. *Clin Ther* 2000; **22**(2): 222–230.

Melki V *et al*. Improvement of HbA1c and blood glucose stability in IDDM patients treated with lispro insulin analog in external pumps. *Diabetes Care* 1998; **21**(6): 977–982.

Perriello G *et al*. The dawn phenomenon in type 1 (insulin-dependent) diabetes mellitus: magnitude, frequency, variability, and dependency on glucose counterregulation and insulin sensitivity. *Diabetologia* 1991; **34**(1): 21–28.

Pieber TR, Eugene-Jolchine I, Derobert E. Efficacy and safety of HOE 901 versus NPH insulin in patients with type 1 diabetes. The European Study Group of HOE 901 in type 1 diabetes. *Diabetes Care* 2000; **23**(2): 157–162.

Raskin P *et al*. Use of insulin aspart, a fast-acting insulin analog, as the mealtime insulin in the management of patients with type 1 diabetes. *Diabetes Care* 2000; **23**(5): 583–588.

Raskin P *et al*. A comparison of insulin lispro and buffered regular human insulin administered via continuous subcutaneous insulin infusion pump. *J Diabetes Complications* 2001; **15**(6): 295–300.

Raskin P *et al*. A 16-week comparison of the novel insulin analog insulin glargine (HOE 901) and NPH human insulin used with insulin lispro in patients with type 1 diabetes. *Diabetes Care* 2000; **23**(11): 1666–1671.

Rosenstock J, Park G, Zimmerman J. Basal insulin glargine (HOE 901) versus NPH insulin in patients with type 1 diabetes on multiple daily insulin regimens. U.S. Insulin Glargine (HOE 901) Type 1 Diabetes Investigator Group. *Diabetes Care* 2000; **23**(8): 1137–1142.

Rosenstock J *et al*. Basal insulin therapy in type 2 diabetes: 28-week comparison of insulin glargine (HOE 901) and NPH insulin. *Diabetes Care* 2001; **24**(4): 631–636.

Yki-Jarvinen H. Combination therapy with insulin and oral agents: optimizing glycemic control in patients with type 2 diabetes mellitus. *Diabetes Metab Res Rev* 2002; **18**(Suppl 3): S77–S81.

Appendix 1 – Drugs

Oral antihyperglycaemic drugs

Drug	Trade name *not UK	Preparation	Strength	Doses used to lower blood glucose (adult)	Comments	Side effects
Sulphonylureas						
Glibenclamide (glyburide)	Daonil Diabeta*	Tablet	5 mg	2.5–10 mg prior to breakfast and evening meal or 2.5–15 mg with breakfast	Contraindicated in severe hepatic and renal impairment, porphyria, pregnancy (substitute insulin), breast feeding, elderly (use shorter acting sulphonylurea); caution in mild to moderate hepatic and renal impairment	Hypoglycaemia; gastrointestinal disturbances (nausea, vomiting, diarrhoea, constipation), disturbances in hepatic function (cholestatic jaundice, hepatitis), hypersensitivity reactions (mainly allergic skin reactions shortly after starting therapy)
	Semi-Daonil	Tablet	2.5 mg			
	Euglycon	Tablet	2.5, 5 mg			
Glicazide	Diamicron	Tablet	80 mg	40–160 mg prior to breakfast and evening meal	Contraindicated in severe hepatic and renal impairment, porphyria, pregnancy (substitute insulin), breast feeding; caution in mild to moderate hepatic and renal impairment	Hypoglycaemia – less than seen with glibenclamide; gastrointestinal disturbances (nausea, vomiting, diarrhoea, constipation), disturbances in hepatic function (cholestatic jaundice, hepatitis), hypersensitivity reactions (mainly allergic skin reactions shortly after starting therapy)
	Diamicron MR	M/R tablet	30 mg	30 mg with breakfast (max 120 mg/d)		
Glimepiride	Amaryl	Tablet	1, 2, 3, 4 mg	1 mg/d before or with breakfast, range 1–4 mg/d (max 8 mg)	Contraindicated in severe hepatic and renal impairment, porphyria, pregnancy (substitute insulin), breast feeding, elderly (use shorter acting sulphonylurea); caution in mild to moderate hepatic and renal impairment	Hypoglycaemia, gastrointestinal disturbances (nausea, vomiting, diarrhoea, constipation), disturbances in hepatic function (cholestatic jaundice, hepatitis), hypersensitivity reactions (mainly allergic skin reactions shortly after starting therapy)

Oral antihyperglycaemic drugs (continued)

Drug	Trade name	Preparation	Strength	Doses used to lower blood glucose (adult)	Comments	Side effects
Sulphonylureas						
Glipizide	Glibenese	Tablet	5 mg	2.5–5 mg before-breakfast, (max single dose 15 mg, divided dose 20 mg/d)	Contraindicated in severe hepatic and renal impairment, porphyria, pregnancy (substitute insulin), breast feeding, elderly (use shorter acting sulphonylurea); caution in mild to moderate hepatic and renal impairment	Gastrointestinal disturbances (nausea, vomiting, diarrhoea, constipation), disturbances in hepatic function (cholestatic jaundice, hepatitis), hypersensitivity reactions (mainly allergic skin reactions shortly after starting therapy), dizziness, drowsiness
	Minodiab	Tablet	2.5, 5 mg			
Gliquidone	Glurenorm	Tablet	30 mg	15 mg before break-fast increasing to 45–60 mg/d in 2 or 3 divided doses (max single dose 60 mg, divided dose 180 mg/d)	Contraindicated in severe hepatic and renal impairment, porphyria, pregnancy (substitute insulin), breast feeding, elderly (use shorter acting sulphonylurea); caution in mild to moderate hepatic and renal impairment	Gastrointestinal disturbances (nausea, vomiting, diarrhoea, constipation), disturbances in hepatic function (cholestatic jaundice, hepatitis), hypersensitivity reactions (mainly allergic skin reactions shortly after starting therapy), headache, tinnitus
Tolbutamide	Generic	Tablet	500 mg	0.5–1.5 g/d with or immediately after breakfast (max 2 g/d in divided doses)	Contraindicated in severe hepatic and renal impairment, porphyria, pregnancy (substitute insulin), breast feeding; caution in mild to moderate hepatic and renal impairment	Gastrointestinal disturbances (nausea, vomiting, diarrhoea, constipation), disturbances in hepatic function (cholestatic jaundice, hepatitis), hypersensitivity reactions (mainly allergic skin reactions shortly after starting therapy)

Oral antihyperglycaemic drugs (continued)

Drug	Trade name *not UK	Preparation	Strength	Doses used to lower blood glucose (adult)	Comments	Side effects
Biguanide – decreased hepatic glucose output						
Metformin	Glucophage	Tablet	500, 850 mg	500 mg before evening meal increasing after 1 week to 500 mg before breakfast and evening meal and then 500 mg before breakfast, lunch and evening meal and bedtime prn (usual max 2.5 g/d)	Most suitable drug for obese patients when dieting has failed to control diabetes; contraindicated in hepatic and renal impairment, predisposition to lactic acidosis, ketoacidosis, heart failure, severe infection and trauma, dehydration, alcohol dependence, pregnancy, breast feeding; does not cause hypoglycaemia	Gastrointestinal disturbances (anorexia, nausea, vomiting, diarrhoea), abdominal pain, metallic taste, lactic acidosis – rare, decreased vitamin B12 absorption
Alpha glucosidase inhibitor						
Acarbose	Glucobay Prandase*	Tablet	50, 100 mg	25–50 mg/d increasing to 50 mg 3 times/d then 100 mg 3 times/d after 6–8 weeks prn (max 200 mg 3 times daily); swallow whole immediately before first bite of food	Contraindicated in inflammatory bowel diseases (Crohn's disease, ulcerative colitis), partial intestinal obstruction, hepatic impairment, severe renal impairment, hernia, history of abdominal surgery, pregnancy, breast feeding	Flatulence, soft stools, diarrhoea (tends to decrease with time), abdominal distention and pain, abnormal liver function tests, skin reactions, ileus, oedema, jaundice, hepatitis; does not cause hypoglycaemia

Oral antihyperglycaemic drugs (continued)

Drug	Trade name *not UK	Preparation	Strength	Doses used to lower blood glucose (adult)	Comments	Side effects
Fast-acting insulin secretagogues						
Nateglinide	Starlix	Tablet	60, 120, 180 mg	60 mg 3 times/d before main meals (max 180 mg 3 times/d)	Contraindicated in diabetic ketoacidosis, severe hepatic impairment, pregnancy and breast feeding; caution in debilitated and malnourished patients, moderate hepatic impairment, substitute insulin during intercurrent illness and surgery; tablets can be withheld with missed meals	Hypoglycaemia – less than with sulphonylureas; hypersensitivity reactions (pruritus, rashes, urticaria)
Repaglinide	NovoNorm Gluconorm*	Tablet	500 µg, 1 mg, 2 mg	1 mg before main meals (max single dose 4 mg, max divided dose 16 mg/d)	Contraindicated in diabetic ketoacidosis, severe hepatic impairment, pregnancy and breast feeding; caution in debilitated and malnourished patients, renal impairment, substitute insulin during intercurrent illness and surgery; tablets can be withheld with missed meals	Hypoglycaemia – less than with sulphonylureas; abdominal pain, diarrhoea, constipation, nausea, vomiting, hypersensitivity reactions (pruritus, rashes, urticaria)

Oral antihyperglycaemic drugs (continued)

Drug	Trade name	Preparation	Strength	Doses used to lower blood glucose (adult)	Comments	Side effects
Thiazolidinediones – insulin sensitizers						
Pioglitazone	Actos	Tablet	15, 30, 45 mg	15–45 mg/d can be taken at anytime of day, irrespective of mealtime	Used in combination with metformin or an insulin stimulating drug; contraindicated in patients with heart failure (due to risk of fluid retention), hepatic impairment, history of heart failure, pregnancy, breast feeding; monitor liver function during treatment; caution in cardiovascular disease	Weight gain, fluid retention, anaemia, gastrointestinal disturbances, headache, visual disturbances, dizziness, arthralgia, haematuria, impotence; does not cause hypoglycaemia
Rosiglitazone	Avandia	Tablet	4, 8 mg	4–8 mg/d can be taken at any time of day irrespective of mealtime	Used in combination with metformin or an insulin stimulating drug; contraindicated in patients with heart failure (due to risk of fluid retention), hepatic impairment, history of heart failure, pregnancy, breast feeding; monitor liver function during treatment; caution in cardiovascular disease, renal impairment	Gastrointestinal disturbances, headache, anaemia, fatigue, weight gain, fluid retention

Insulins

Drug	Trade name * not UK	Preparation	Time action	Comments	Side effects
Analogue fast-acting					
Aspart	NovoRapid	Vial: Penfill; FlexPen; NovoLet	10–120 minutes	Taken immediately prior to any meal or major snack; provides increased flexibility; variation of dose with differing meals and activities; less hypoglycaemia	Hypoglycaemia
Lispro	Humalog	Vial: Autopen; HumaPen; Humalog-Pen	10–120 minutes	Taken immediately prior to any meal or major snack; provides increased flexibility; variation of dose with differing meals and activities; less hypoglycaemia	Hypoglycaemia
Soluble human					
Soluble (human regular)	Actrapid	Vial: Penfill; NovoLet	2–8 hours	Needs to be taken 45–60 minutes before meal; less flexibility	Hypoglycaemia
	Velosulin	Vial			
	Humulin S	Vial: Autopen; HumaPen; Humaject S			
	Humulin R*	Vial: Penfill			
	Insuman Rapid	Vial: OptiPen Pro: Rapid OptiSet			
	Toronto*	Vial: Penfill			

Insulins (continued)

Drug	Trade name *not UK	Preparation	Time action	Comments	Side effects
Intermediate (basal)					
Isophane (NPH)	Insulatard	Vial; Penfill; FlexPen; NovoLet; InnoLet	2–12 hours	Taken at bedtime: bedtime/prebreakfast	Hypoglycaemia
	Humulin I	Vial: Autopen; HumaPen; Humulin I-Pen			
	Insuman Basal	Vial: OptiPen Pro; OptiSet			
	Novolin NPH*	Vial; Penfill			
	Humulin N*	Vial; Penfill			
Zinc suspension (lente)	Monotard	Vial	2–12 hours	taken at bedtime: bedtime/prebreakfast	Hypoglycaemia
	Humulin Lente	Vial			
Long acting					
Zinc suspension crystalline (ultra-lente)	Ultratard	Vial	16–36 hours	Definite peak; absorption irregular, exact time action varies	Hypoglycaemia
	Humulin Zn	Vial			
Glargine	Lantus	Vial: OptiPen Pro; OptiSet	4–24 hours	Taken at bedtime; peakless longer-acting insulin; less nocturnal hypoglycaemia	Hypoglycaemia

Insulins (continued)

Drug	Trade name	Preparation	Time action	Comments	Side effects
Biphasic (mixed)					
Aspart/aspart protamine	NovoMix 30	Penfill; FlexPen	10 minutes to 24 hours	Taken immediately prior to breakfast and evening meal	Hypoglycaemia
Lispro/lispro protamine	Humalog Mix25	Autopen; HumaPen; prefilled disposable injection devices	10 minutes to 24 hours	Taken immediately prior to breakfast and evening meal	Hypoglycaemia
	Humalog Mix50	Prefilled disposable injection devices			
Soluble/isophane (regular/NPH)	Mixtard 10	Penfill; NovoLet	2–24 hours	Needs to be taken 45–60 minutes before meal	Hypoglycaemia
	Mixtard 20	Penfill; NovoLet			
	Mixtard 30	Vial; Penfill; NovoLet; InnoLet			
	Mixtard 40	Penfill; NovoLet			
	Mixtard 50	Penfill; NovoLet			
	Humulin M2	Autopen; HumaPen			
	Humulin M3	Vial; Autopen; HumaPen; Humaject			
	Humulin M5	Vial			
	Insuman Comb 15	Vial; OptiPen; OptiSet			
	Insuman Comb 25	Vial; OptiPen; OptiSet			
	Insuman Comb 50	Vial; OptiPen; OptiSet			

Appendix 2 – Useful Addresses and Websites

For the physician
Societies

American Diabetes Association
Address: (Attn: National Call Center), 1701 North Beauregard Street, Alexandria, VA 22311, USA
Tel.: (800) 342 2383
Website: http://www.diabetes.org

British Association of Retinal Screeners
Website: http://www.eyescreening.org.uk/home.html

British Cardiac Society
Address: 9 Fitzroy Square, London W1T 5HW, UK
Tel.: 0207 383 3887
Fax: 0207 388 0903
E-mail: enquiries@bcs.com
Website: http://www.bcs.com

British Dietetic Association
Address: 5th Floor, Charles House, 148/9 Great Charles Street Queensway, Birmingham B3 3HT, UK
Tel.: 0121 200 8080
Fax: 0121 200 8081
E-mail: info@bda.uk.com
Website: http://www.bda.uk.com

British Hypertension Society
E-mail: bhsis@sghms.ac.uk
Website: http://www.hyp.ac.uk/bhs

British Society for Paediatric Endocrinology and Diabetes
Website: http://www.bsped.org.uk

Canadian Diabetes Association
Website: http://www.diabetes.ca/Section_Main/welcome.asp

Clinical Guidelines 2003:
http://www.diabetes.ca/cpg2003/chapters.aspx

Guidelines on Hypoglycaemia:
http://www.diabetes.ca/Section_Main/NewsReleases.asp?ID=37

Canadian Hypertension Society
Recommendations and teaching slides:
http://www.chs.md/index2.html

Canadian Lipid Guidelines
Website: http://www.cmaj.ca/cgi/content/full/169/9/921

Diabetes Network International
E-mail: info@dni.org.uk
Website: http://www.dni.org.uk

European Association for the Study of Diabetes
Address: Rheindorfer Weg 3, D-40591 Dusseldorf, Germany
Tel.: +49-211 75 84 69-0
Fax: +49-211 75 84 69 29
E-mail: secretariat@easd.org
Website: http://www.easd.org

Primary Care Diabetes UK
Address: 10 Parkway, London NW1 7AA, UK
Tel.: 0207 424 1000
Fax: 0207 424 1001
E-mail: info@diabetes.org.uk
Website: http://www.diabetes.org.uk/home.htm

Journals

British Journal of Diabetes & Vascular Disease
http://www.bjdvd.co.uk
Diabetic Medicine
http://www.blackwell-science.com/dme

For the patient
Societies

American Diabetes Association
Address: (Attn: National Call Center), 1701 North Beauregard
Street, Alexandria, VA 22311, USA
Tel.: (800) 342 2383
Website: http://www.diabetes.org

British Heart Foundation
Address: 14 Fitzhardinge Street, London W1H 6DH, UK
Tel.: 0207 935 0185
Fax: 0207 486 5820
E-mail: internet@bhf.org.uk
Website: http://www.bhf.org.uk

Canadian Diabetes Association
Website: http://www.diabetes.ca/Section_Main/welcome.asp

Diabetes UK
Address: 10 Parkway, London NW1 7AA, UK
Tel.: 0207 424 1000
Fax: 0207 424 1001
E-mail: info@diabetes.org.uk
Website: http://www.diabetes.org.uk/home.htm
Careline: 0845 120 2960

Index

Note: Page numbers followed by 'f' and 't' indicate figures and tables respectively. This index is presented in letter-by-letter order, whereby spaces and hyphens in main entries are excluded by the alphabetization process. As diabetes is the subject of the book, all index entries refer to diabetes unless otherwise indicated.